Student Study Guide for Breastfeeding and Human Lactation

KATHLEEN G. AUERBACH
JAN RIORDAN

Jones and Bartlett Publishers
Boston London

Editorial, Sales, and Customer Services offices:
Jones and Bartlett Publishers
One Exeter Plaza
Boston, MA 02116

Jones and Bartlett Publishers International
PO Box 1498
London W6 7RS
England

ISBN: 0-86720-632-2

Printed in the United States of America
97   96   95   94   93   10   9   8   7   6   5   4   3   2   1

TABLE OF CONTENTS

GUIDELINES FOR USING THE STUDY GUIDE

This Study Guide, which accompanies the reference textbook *Breastfeeding and Human Lactation* is designed to assist both the learner and the teacher in the study of breastfeeding/lactation. For the learner, we designed this Study Guide to help you assess your current knowledge and/or to help you prepare for certification as a lactation consultant. For the teacher, we are providing basic tools for developing a lactation course, whether it is presented with a classical academic orientation or with an emphasis on clinical skills. The user of this Study Guide is referred to the textbook for preparation for proceeding through the Study Guide–whether the reader's intent is to gain an understanding about breastfeeding and lactation issues, to prepare to take a certification examination in the field of lactation, or to self-test her or his own level of knowledge and understanding of the lactation process.

The Study Guide is organized to correspond to the progression of chapters in Breastfeeding and Human Lactation. Each chapter in this Study Guide contains the following:

- Outline of the corresponding chapter in the reference textbook
- Key concepts which highlight the concepts stressed in corresponding chapter
- Multiple-choice questions which test the learner's level of understanding of certain facts about lactation and breastfeeding; after answering these questions, the learner may compare her/his answers to the correct answers listed on page 123.
- Short-answer questions which may or may not have "one correct" answer, but which are designed to spark discussions among learners
- Essay questions which can be used for course examinations or to stimulate class discussion
- Story problems which present advanced students with a scenario that requires them to integrate knowledge from several disciplines and to delineate actions based upon this synthesis.

We recommend that the last three items listed above be used for group work.

Since there is no one right answer, but rather a probable answer depending upon how the student has chosen to handle the situation, these questions are ideal for inductive learning, whereby several peers participate in solving problems and thus learn from one another's experience. The reference textbook was written to be used at both the undergraduate and graduate levels. However, since graduate study is organized so that experienced practitioners share knowledge and solve problems collectively, these last three items especially lend themselves to use in graduate-level programs.

We expect that instructors teaching a lactation course may find the textbook too long for a one-semester course. While each teacher will want to select chapters that meet students' learning needs and specific course objectives, we anticipate that most instructors using the textbook will choose to assign major sections of Chapters 4, 5, 6, 9, 13, 14, 18, and 19 for the first level of the course and the remaining chapters for the second level.

Some Comments on the Study Exercises

The set of multiple-choice and true/false questions help you to assess level of learning. If you selected the correct answers, congratulations! You recall what you have read and are now in a better position to use that new knowledge in your daily work. If you selected an incorrect answer, try to determine where you went wrong and–most important–why you did so. Perhaps you misread the question. Perhaps you read only a portion of the question and the options that followed, thereby selecting a "distractor" that was partially correct, but not the one best answer. Perhaps you simply did not know the right response. If you answered incorrectly, go back and reread the question and the correct answer. Ask yourself, "Do I understand why the authors say that is the correct answer?" If you do not understand how the correct answer relates to the question, go back to the chapter from which the question was derived and reread that portion pertaining to the question.

After you have tested your new knowledge about the facts relating to breastfeeding and lactation, you will want to go on to the essay questions and the story problems. The essay questions give you an opportunity to explain–in your own words–your understanding of not just the facts, but how several pieces of information relate to one another and thus affect behavior or experience. We have not provided answers to these questions because such answers, while based in part on the information provided in *Breastfeeding and Human Lactation*, may go beyond the material in the textbook to take into account your experiences as well. Thus, in checking your answers to the short-answer questions and the essay questions, please refer to the textbook, but also permit a degree of latitude based on life experience and/or discussion with colleagues.

Likewise, when you work through the story problems, there is no one right answer, but rather a series of probable answers, depending on how you handle the situation. Make the best use of the story problems by attempting to answer each one. Do not skip a problem–such as one relating to Chapter 21 (Research and Breastfeeding)–because you do not feel the issues apply to you. Each health-care worker asks and answers research questions every day–every time a client presents a particular problem and you select from a variety of options a care plan that you consider optimal for that client. We recommend that you work with your colleagues when using the story problems. Perhaps one could be the focus for a journal club meeting that is reviewing a particular article or series of articles. Or, if your clinical service has a weekly meeting to discuss a particular case, ask if you might present a hypothetical case that raises issues similar to those you faced with a client; use the questions from a particular story problem to generate discussion.

Remember, when you answer the multiple-choice and short-answer essay questions, you are demonstrating that you know certain facts about lactation and breastfeeding. When you answer the essay questions and story problems, you are demonstrating that you can draw on that knowledge to frame responses to questions you are likely to encounter in the "real" world of lactation consulting. In short, you are testing–if you use the questions provided in this Study Guide–your cognitive knowledge as well as your ability to use that information in an insightful and creative manner.

We recommend that you use this Study Guide as one means of learning about lactation and breastfeeding. While you may read each chapter of the textbook from which these questions are derived and study alone part of the time, we recommend that you go over the questions and discuss the answers with two or more of your peers who are also preparing for lactation certification and/or who are already working in the field. In this manner, all of you can gain from the unique strengths of one another. Also, role-playing the story problems may help each of you to see how varying answers can lead one in different directions, requiring altered emphasis to particular concerns.

In addition to learning situations, this Study Guide will serve as a resource by providing recent references that back up recommendations on optimal breastfeeding management. It may also be used for research endeavors since it highlights questions requiring research-generated answers–as well as a guide to both the current knowledge and practices in the field of lactation. (See especially the clinical implications in each chapter.)

PREPARING FOR THE CERTIFICATION EXAMINATION IN LACTATION

A certification examination in lactation/breastfeeding is designed to identify your knowledge of cognitive material and your ability to use that information when confronted with problems of greater or lesser complexity. A certification examination, by its very nature, requires both stamina and patience. You need stamina because the certification exam is likely to be longer than other examinations you have taken. You need patience because the actions of others, namely the administrator of the examination, will control your actions at certain times. More about this later. You will do best if you enter the test situation as relaxed as you can be, ready to demonstrate how much you know. To do this, you need to be able to set aside any anxieties that derive from the testing situation. In this case, knowing something about what you face can help reduce your anxiety. (See the following list for some general test-taking strategies.)

General Test-Taking Strategies

1. Review the material over a period of time. Avoid cramming.
2. Pace yourself when taking sample examinations. Try to answer one question in one minute.
3. Read each question completely and carefully before selecting an answer.
4. Concentrate on the information offered in the question. Do not read information into the question or allow your mind to wander back to previous questions.
5. Select the one option that you think is the best response.
6. If you are unsure, eliminate clearly incorrect options before selecting from the remaining "distractors."
7. Use the answer sheet only to record the single answer you have selected for each question.
8. Use the test booklet to jot notes, eliminate options, and the like.
9. Identify the rationale for each question and answer in terms of that rationale.
10. Use relaxation techniques if you become anxious or tense.

The certification examination sponsored by the International Board of Lactation Consultant Examiners, Inc. (IBLCE) is divided into two separate segments. The morning session is devoted exclusively to multiple-choice questions. The test booklet contains all the information you need to answer each question. You will be asked to record your answers on a separate answer sheet. You are given a set amount of time to answer all of these questions; you may leave the examination room when you have completed this portion of the exam without incurring a penalty. Thus, if you are a quick test-taker, you may find yourself with sufficient time to take a brief nap before lunch and still be able to return to the testing site on time. If you are a slow test-taker, you should still find that you have sufficient time to complete all of the first segment of questions within the time provided. Because your total score is based on the number of correct answers you provide, it is appropriate to engage in educated guessing. You will be allowed to write in your test booklet. Thus, noting which option is clearly wrong, and which ones you aren't sure of, is allowed. However, make sure that your answer sheet includes only one answer for each question.

The afternoon session is reserved for answering multiple-choice questions keyed to the viewing of slide material. It is this segment that can be most troublesome if you are unfamiliar with how such an examination is given. For each slide, a particular time period is provided to answer the multiple-choice question; then the next slide is shown. Practice for this portion beforehand by looking at slides and then answering imaginary questions about them. Doing this can help to reduce your anxiety so that you can concentrate–rather than being distracted by the instructions of the testing administrator, who changes the slides and tells you to go on to the next question.

The goal of the certification examinee is to pass; you need not do so with the top score in order to be certified. Usually the cutoff point between passing and not passing is below 70%. You will help yourself by attempting to answer as many of the questions as possible. If you tend to take tests slowly, practice answering multiple-choice questions with four "distractors" within a set time limit–about one question per minute–in order to increase the speed with which you proceed through the examination questions. Remember: if you finish early, you can always go back over questions about which you were unsure; however, if you proceed too slowly and you have not answered all of the questions when the exam administrator asks you to close your examination booklet, you will have penalized yourself by not moving more quickly through the questions.

Multiple-Choice Questions

Most certification examinations, including the one administered by the IBLCE, consist of a long series (200 or more) of multiple-choice questions. Knowing something about this kind of question will reduce your anxiety about identifying the correct answer, particularly if you have never taken such an examination before. If you have never taken multiple-choice examinations before, you may find the structured nature of the questions difficult to understand. Practicing with the multiple-choice questions provided in this Study Guide may help you to feel more comfortable with this form of test question.

Each question begins with a stem–either a question or the beginning of a statement– followed by three or more options, which are either answers to the question or the completion of the statement. Each question has one best answer mixed in with several options or "distractors." In most cases, choices which are obviously incorrect will be easy to identify. It is your job to ferret out the one best response from among those answers that are partially correct. If you take tests quickly, you may find that the time provided for the examination is far longer than you need. If you tend to take tests slowly, you may feel rushed and frustrated that you cannot set your own speed for a particular portion of the exam, especially the part involving visual material.

However rapidly or slowly you take tests, it is wise to practice ahead of time. Studying with peers can offer you such opportunities. In addition, workshops designed to assist candidates for certification to take "practice" exams may also be available in your area. Take advantage of them: simply gaining familiarity with the manner in which questions are asked will help to reduce your anxiety about being in a testing situation.

After answering several multiple-choice questions from this Study Guide, you can gain additional familiarity with this form of test question by writing some yourself. Giving these questions to your colleagues will not only require you to make sure that your questions are clear, but also that you have provided only ONE BEST answer, rather than a series of partially correct responses. (See the sample test questions based on this material on pages xv–xvi.)

Questions Deriving from Visual Material

Long ago, Plautus (254-184 B.C.) said, "Patience is the best remedy for every trouble." While we doubt that he was thinking about multiple-choice exams, his comment surely applies to that portion of the IBLCE-administered lactation certification exam which gives most candidates the greatest difficulty. We are referring to the slide portion of the test. The speed with which you move through this segment of the exam is controlled by the examination administrator, who has been instructed to provide you with a view of a particular slide for a set period of time (usually 90 seconds). Therefore, in this portion of the examination, you do not have the luxury of returning to a question about which you were unsure. You must identify what you are looking at, read the question pertaining to that material, decide on the best answer to the question, and mark your answer before the examination administrator moves on to the next slide or other piece of visual material. While 90 seconds may seem like a very short period of time, you will probably find that in most cases you have made your selection of the correct answer long before the time period is up.

Your best preparation for the certification examination is methodical studying coupled with creative group discussions for several months in advance of the exam. If you think of the exam as a performance, you will see that regular, frequent rehearsals will prepare you best and add to your confidence. Many successful certification candidates meet with their peers once or twice a week for several months; each is responsible for leading a discussion about a particular aspect of lactation or breastfeeding.

Using *Breastfeeding and Human Lactation* as your textbook, assign a different person or persons to lead a discussion based on a particular chapter. We recommend that all of the study group then go through the questions deriving from the chapter being discussed. Use the multiple-choice questions as a practice session for the certification exam. Use the short-answer questions as the basis for writing additional multiple-choice questions. And use the essay questions and story problems to gain additional understanding of the issues under consideration. Setting aside a set time each day or each week to go through sample test questions will help you more than trying to read one more book two nights before the examination.

The night before the examination, exercise vigorously enough so that you can relax and get a good night's sleep. The next morning, begin the day with a meal that provides both sufficient protein and calories to keep you going for several hours <u>and</u> that sits lightly in your stomach. This is not the time to try out a new recipe or to include an ingredient that gave you gas three years ago! Cramming the night, or a few days, beforehand does not help; instead of preparing you, such activity is more apt to increase your level of anxiety by focusing your attention on what you don't know. Additionally, getting an inadequate amount of sleep the night before reduces your alertness and your ability to think creatively in a stressful situation. Eating a breakfast that is too light–or no breakfast at all–does not provide you with the energy you will need to endure the morning session.

Anxiety

If at any time before or during the exam you feel panicky, take several deep breaths. If you know breathing techniques for labor and childbirth, use them. Close your eyes and try to visualize yourself in a safe and relaxing place. Some test-takers say to themselves, "This is an EASY exam," or "I know most all of the answers," or "I know how to take this kind of exam." Such thoughts help to create a positive mind-set.

Avoid frightening yourself with negative messages, such as "I don't know if I can pass this test," or "I'm going to fail." When studying for the exam, and while taking it, practice progressive relaxation by relaxing successive muscle groups. Begin with the tips of your toes and work upward, or start at the top of your head and work downward.   If you feel your heart beating rapidly, tell yourself, "I am going to breathe deeply and my heart rate will slow." Then imagine your heart slowing as you breathe deeply and slowly several times. If you practice these exercises before you take the exam, you will find yourself able to relax while you are in the examination.

No one has yet expired from taking a certification exam. Ideally, you will enter the examination room alert to your surroundings and ready to concentrate on the task at hand. It is okay to feel a bit anxious, but you do not want such anxiety to interfere with your ability to demonstrate what you know. Think of the exam as a series of hurdles of varying heights, most of which will be so low that you can simply sail over them without breaking stride! Each time you answer a question, you have cleared another of those hurdles. In doing so, you will gain confidence that most of the rest of those hurdles will not cause you to trip and fall. If you encounter a series of questions that are confusing to you–or that you simply haven't any idea how to answer–go on to the next question that you can answer, making sure that you place your answer to that question in the correctly numbered space on your answer sheet. When you have finished the rest of the questions, you should have time to go back to the pesky set that initially threw you.

Approach each question as if it were the only thing you cared about. Begin your assault on the question by reading it through completely. The mistake quick test-takers make most often is partially reading a question and selecting an answer on the basis of incomplete information. After you have read through the entire question, look for words that give you a clue as to incorrect "distractors." Words like "always" and "never" will rarely be part of a correct answer. Identifying clearly incorrect "distractors" first is a good way to begin if you have to guess, or you are eliminating certain "distractors." Remember, too, that your first guess is usually the right one. Trust your intuition, "best judgment," or whatever you call a hunch. However, do not hurt yourself by making wild guesses or by trying to figure out how many times item a, but not item b, will be correct.

If you encounter a question that completely stumps you, go on to others and come back to that one. Your unconscious may discern the answer to the "toughy" while you are concentrating on other items.

Avoid changing answers. Very often, you will change a correct answer to an incorrect one, particularly if you are inclined to "read into" a question. It is rarely wise to try to "second-guess" possible writer(s) of the question; in most cases, several individuals have contributed to each question.

Once you have completed a question, try to put it out of your mind. Your job now is to answer the next item. Do not dwell on a question that was bothersome or a stem that made no sense to you. Such mulling will simply waste time you need to correctly answer the other questions.

For best results, follow the general rules found in the following list–both when you practice taking a multiple-choice examination and when you take the certification examination.

Key Guidelines for Taking a Multiple-Choice Examination

1. Look for priority questions that ask for first or last actions, choices, and the like. While all the choices offered may be correct actions, the highest priority response is usually the one best answer.
2. If a lengthy situation or a slide or other visual material is provided, look at the question stem first. This will give you a clue regarding what information is being sought.
3. Watch for negative words and prefixes—for example, "All of the following are true except." Decide on the direction of the stem (positive/negative) before proceeding with the question.
4. Select the response you best understand.
5. Trust your intuition; trust yourself. Your first hunch is usually the right answer.
6. Pace yourself. Try to complete each question within one minute. Your score will be higher if you have guessed at some questions and you finish the test rather than if you complete only a portion of the exam and all your answers are correct.

Snacks and Medicines

Physical discomfort, such as hunger, detracts from being able to concentrate on the examination. If you are allowed to bring hard candies or other munchables with you, do so. When you are struggling to think through a particularly knotty question, a bit of quick energy may be just the thing to help you relax. If you are taking the examination in the middle of a sinusitis attack, a cold, or other condition that causes you periodic discomfort, do not take a remedy, such as an antihistamine, beforehand; it may cause drowsiness.

Sites

Examination sites differ. You may be asked to report to a hotel room, which may or may not have windows. You may be in a college or university lecture room which is more conducive to taking an examination. Or you may be in a large church hall or other public space which has never been used in quite this manner before. People who are not test-takers may be making distracting noise outside the room. Lights may make the slide portion of the exam hard to see. If this is the case, ask your examination administrator to make the appropriate adjustments.

Clothing

Regardless of the season of the year, it is best to dress in layers so that if the room is warm, you can remove some outer clothing in order to remain comfortable. Assume that at least part of the time you will feel too cold. This may be caused by air-conditioning, a draft from a window or fan, or by your own anxiety. Hotel conference rooms in the United States are notorious for being cold, almost to the point of being uninhabitable. A sweater or jacket over other clothing will keep you from being so chilled that you cannot concentrate on the task at hand.

The Exam is Over!

When you have completed the examination, celebrate having survived–and then try to forget about it. It will be many weeks before you learn how well you did. Until the day you receive your certificate identifying you as a certified lactation consultant, concentrate on the rest of your busy and fulfilling life.

SAMPLE TEST QUESTIONS

Use the following test questions to practice some of the techniques discussed in the preceding pages.

1. The most effective technique for using a textbook to study for an exam is to:
    a. read the textbook as close to the exam date as possible
    b. read the textbook a little at a time
    c. use the questions in the Study Guide to test knowledge of the textbook
    d. b and c above
    e. all of the above

- Distractor a is clearly incorrect. Following its advice is likely to increase your anxiety and prevent you from getting through the material in advance of the exam!
- Distractor b is good advice, particularly when you are attempting to learn and remember a large body of information–just as small meals that are well digested are more easily swallowed than large meals wolfed down.
- Distractor c is also good advice. The Study Guide is designed to highlight important aspects of each chapter. Using the questions in the Study Guide can help you to remember those items that are most likely to be used as the basis for test questions.
- Distractor d is the one best answer. Why? Because it includes both of the options that are, by themselves, partially correct.
- Distractor e is incorrect. Why? Because it includes an obviously incorrect distractor along with the correct ones. Therefore, it is not the one best answer.

2. When confronted by a multiple-choice question you do not understand:
    a. select the most difficult-to-understand distractor
    b. go back to the question later

c.   select the one option you do understand
d.   guess at the answer any way you wish

- Distractor a is a poor choice. The less you understand, the less likely you are to select the correct answer.
- Distractor b is a better choice. Time, relaxing a bit more, and getting into a test-taking mode may be all you need to understand the question more completely.
- Distractor c is the best choice. The option you understand is more likely than others to be the correct answer. Remember: the test writers are <u>not</u> trying to trick you.
- Distractor d is a poor choice. Guessing might be all right if you have reduced your choices down to two; this at least gives you a 50-50 chance of guessing correctly. However, guessing from four options gives you only a 25% chance of correctly answering the question. You want to improve your odds before guessing.

3. When you are taking a multiple-choice test that includes slide material, how should you approach the question?
    a.   look at the slide for at least 30 seconds and then read the question
    b.   read the stem of the question first; look at the slide; then read the options
    c.   read the stem of the question and all of the options; then look at the slide
    d.   look at the slide and then read the options

- Distractor a is a poor choice. Simply looking at the slide for a long period may not tell you what is being asked for. You may lose valuable time following this advice.
- Distractor b is a good choice. By reading the stem of the question, you may be given a clue as to what to look for in the visual material. This will help you select the options.
- Distractor c is a poor choice. If you spend too much time on the written portion of the question, you may not have enough time to examine the visual material.
- Distractor d is also a poor choice. The slide material may, in the absence of awareness of the stem, give you an incorrect impression when selecting the options.

In question 3, the choices may seem less clear-cut, but there is still <u>one best</u> answer–distractor b. Use this technique when you practice viewing slide materials for which multiple-choice questions have been prepared.

SECTION

ONE

Historical and Sociocultural Context of Infant Feeding

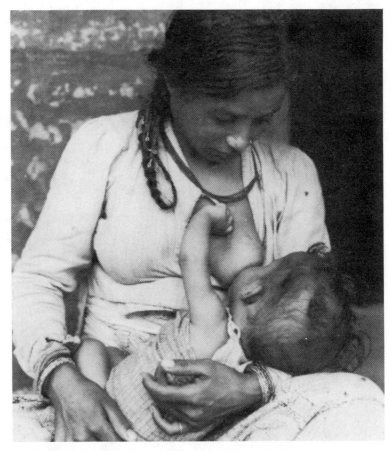

A Nepalese mother provides her baby with the best start in life. (Photo by Jack Ling/UNICEF)

1

Tides in Breastfeeding Practice

1: Outline

2: List of Key Concepts in the Chapter

The reader is urged to look for these key concepts in the body of the chapter and to develop questions deriving from these concepts as one way to gain understanding and insight into their relationship to lactation and breastfeeding. In this chapter, the reader may find it helpful to compare two different cultures of which s/he is familiar, noting specific beliefs that influence behaviors and attitudes relating to breastfeeding and/or lactation–including its promotion and management, as well as when and how long women are expected to breastfeed.

Breastfeeding practices
Breastfeeding promotion
Breastfeeding regulation
Hand-feeding
Infant mortality
Manufactured baby milks
Mixed feeds
Pre-lacteal feeds
Wet-nursing
WHO Code
WIC Program

3: Multiple-Choice Questions

1. Over the last 50 years:
    a. more babies are being breastfed than 50 years ago
    b. about the same percentage of babies are being breastfed, but people in different socioeconomic/ethnic groups are doing so
    c. fewer babies are being breastfed than 50 years ago
    d. more babies are being breastfed in the developing world than 50 years ago, but fewer babies are being breastfed in the developed world

2. Which of the following breastfeeding patterns typifies what is thought to have occurred among human groups before 10,000 B.C.?
    a. frequent breastfeeding
    b. long duration of breastfeeding (more than two years)
    c. infrequent breastfeeding caused by the absence of mother while gathering food
    d. a and b above
    e. b and c above

3. The practice of giving food other than human milk to infants appears to have existed since:
   a. 2000 B.C.
   b. 1000 A.D.
   c. 1500 A.D.
   d. 1850 A.D. to the present

4. During the Industrial Revolution, high infant mortality in countries was linked to:
   a. high breastfeeding rates among those families most likely to breastfeed
   —b. low breastfeeding rates among those families most likely to breastfeed
   c. poverty among those families most likely to breastfeed
   d. a and c above
   e. b and c above

4: Short-Answer Questions

1. Define what the author means by "the range of 'normal' breastfeeding practices" and how that relates to current breastfeeding management. Use two examples to illustrate your understanding of "normal breastfeeding."

2. What is "wet-nursing"? Explain why, in many developed settings, it is rarely practiced today.
   ↓ moral behav. of w.N's

3. What is "hand-feeding"? Identify three different forms of hand-fed foods and note their likely effect on the health/well-being of the infants who receive them.
   liquids, grains, etc. in place of breastmilk — died.
   animal milks, cereals, gruel

4. Explain pre-lacteal feeds. Offer at least three different explanations for their use in different cultures at different time periods.
   Now: Delayed 1st feed + P-L H₂O or ABM feeds,
   neonate feed prior to - in place of colostrum
   cultural taboo-colostrum   1st feed Rx by Dr's

5. Explain why some investigators have concluded that when birth is strictly regulated, breastfeeding rates decline.
   Authority

6. Some writers have placed most of the blame for the use of proprietary baby milks on the drug companies that manufacture and distribute the product. Others blame physicians for attempting to replace that which nature already provides. Select which group you will defend and convince your colleagues that:
   a. Proprietary baby milks are a necessity in a postindustrial society OR
   b. Science can improve upon nature OR
   c. The value of human milk is less important today than it was prior to the Industrial Revolution.

What have you learned from this exercise?

7. What is the relationship between:
   a. artificial feeding and infant health?
   b. declining infant mortality and breastfeeding rates?

8. Identify and briefly discuss four different health risks resulting from the use of artificial baby milks. Explain why some health risks appear to be short-term, while others are long-term.

9. Some investigators contend that when families can afford to artificially feed an infant, it should be their choice to do so. Present a brief, but clear, argument showing how the cost of artificial feeding for a single family also represents costs for the community and society in which that family lives. Use one example from a developing country and one example from a developed country to support your argument.

10. What is the WHO Code and why is it important in a developing country and in a developed country?

5: Essay Questions

1. The author suggests that two conditions are required for women to choose foods other than human milk for their infants: alternative foods must be available, and the use of those foods must be socially acceptable. Identify three different cultural groups.
   a. Explain what foods they use for infants.
   b. Provide examples that support the notion that those foods are acceptable for infants.
   c. Indicate the health risks/benefits derived from the use of those alternative foods within each cultural group selected.

2. Using any developed country as an example, explain how each of the following factors influence breastfeeding initiation and duration:
   a. Women's aspirations in the community and business world
   b. Women's roles relative to men's roles
   c. The availability of alternative infant foods
   d. The usual way in which childbirth is managed
   e. The usual way in which breastfeeding is managed

3.   Explain the role of advertising in the distribution and selling of artificial baby milks. Give examples of three different ways in which these products are advertised–to the public and to health-care professionals.

4.   Identify how class differences in both a developed country and a developing country have influenced the likelihood of breastfeeding initiation and its duration. If the patterns of behavior are different, how do you explain this difference?

5.   Define breastfeeding promotion and provide three different examples of how breastfeeding might be promoted.

6: Story Problem

You are one of a team of scientists (including an anthropologist, a geographer, a botanist, an agricultural specialist, and you, a specialist in infant feeding) in an area where indigenous people live. You must determine how the pattern of infant feeding relates to the totality of this population's way of life.

1.   What are you most interested in observing before you begin to interview your subjects? Why have you selected these elements to observe and what will they tell you?

The people you are observing use a language unfamiliar to you. You cannot get any closer than 10 feet without threatening their "personal space."

2.   How do you continue to gain insight into the infant feeding patterns of these people?

In the course of their own evaluations of these indigenous people, your scientific colleagues leave you near the camp to collect their own data. One afternoon, after exploring a graveyard, you sit down to rest beneath a large tree. You are wakened from your impromptu nap by a gentle tap on your wrist. You look up and find yourself staring into the deep brown eyes of a small child, who scampers back to the safety of his mother's skirt. She smiles at you, and does not move away when you approach.

3.   How do you let her know that you mean no harm–and that you wish to know how she feeds her children?

Two months later, your colleagues return from their wanderings, pleased to discover that you are now accepted by the indigenous group as a harmless oddity in strange dress. Prior to the scientific team's departure, each of you shares what you have learned with the team.

4. What do you tell them about the following?
    a. when mothers initiate breastfeeding, when they do not, and the duration of breastfeeding
    b. whether and for how long they breastfeed exclusively
    c. the mixed feeds that are used and how they are prepared
    d. the overall health status of the children and their mothers
    e. the role of women in the indigenous group
    f. the relationship between women's work and infant care

2

The Cultural Context
of Breastfeeding

1: Outline of the Chapter

Definitions and characteristics
The dominant culture
Assessing culture
Language barriers
The effects of culture on breastfeeding
    Rituals
    Colostrum
    Resuming sexual relations
    Wet-nursing
Childbirth practices
Infant care
Maternal foods
    Foods that increase breastmilk
    Food restrictions
    Vegetarians
    Religious influences
    The "doula"
Weaning
Implications for practice

2: List of Key Concepts in the Chapter

The reader is urged to look for these key concepts in the body of the chapter and to develop questions deriving from these concepts as one way to gain understanding and insight into their relationship to lactation and breastfeeding. In this chapter, the reader is encouraged to examine her/his own cultural heritage in light of attitudes and beliefs that underpin breastfeeding patterns. How amenable to change are those attitudes and beliefs? And, whether or not problems arise, how might new knowledge be incorporated into the culture?

Allopathic medicine
Childbirth
Colostrum
Cultural relativism
Ethnocentrism
Food restrictions
Galactogogues
Infant care
Language
Maternal foods
Milk contamination
Religious Influences
Rituals
Vegetarianism *6+ grains   3+ Veg (+ green)   1-4 fruit (citrus)   milk eggs + allergy*
Weaning
Wet-nursing

3: Multiple-Choice Questions

1. Cultural relativism refers to:
   a. a belief that one's own culture is the only right way in which to live
   b. an appreciation of one's relatives and how they live and work
   c. an appreciation and acceptance of the validity of different cultural systems
   d. b and c above

2. A ritual:
   a. may involve ceremony
   b. may reflect belief in the efficacy of a particular action
   c. has been proven to have positive results
   d. all of the above
   e. a and b above

3. In virtually all cultures meat:
   a. plays a major role in the diet of the pregnant woman
   b. plays a major role in the diet of the lactating woman
   c. usually means beef
   d. none of the above
   e. all of the above
   most cultures - meat minor · flavoring rice, beans + veg.
   major role in Western industrialized countries

4. A galactogogue refers to:
    a. any article of clothing that covers the mammary gland
    b. any food believed to increase milk secretion
    c. any food believed to dry up a mother's milk
    d. any drug that alters galactose

5. Deliberative weaning is practiced: *⇒ by infant development cues*
    a. in nearly all cultures around the world
    b. only in highly developed technological societies
    c. only in the developing world when the mother becomes pregnant again
    d. in those cultures where breastfeeding is considered appropriate only for a
        few months
    e. c and d above

4: Short-Answer Questions

1. What is culture?

2. Briefly distinguish between allopathic and folk medicine. Give an example of a
    belief that typifies each.   *"professional" healthcare*

3. Explain how you might use a focus group to identify beliefs about breastfeeding
    and how to use this information to develop a breastfeeding promotion program
    that is relevant to the target population you have selected.

4. How might knowledge of a "superfood" in a particular culture color your
    approach to encouraging breastfeeding?

5. In what way does language reflect cultural beliefs?

non-product issues = fertility, m satisfaction, bonding, part of maternal experience

6. How might viewing breastfeeding as a process–rather than viewing breastmilk
    as a product–result in different attitudes?   *culture ⇒ process ⇒ few supplements / product ⇒ emph on characteristics (immunal + nutritional)*

7. For each of the following, provide an example of a positive outcome and a
    negative outcome, each of which helps to explain how culture influences the
    behavior in question:
    a. childbirth
    b. sexual relations
    c. breastfeeding
    d. wet-nursing
    e. swaddling

8. How might a 40-day (six-week) period of seclusion after childbirth assist the mother? *estab lactation + bonding*

9. Briefly explain why "evil eye" is almost never a diagnosis offered to explain infant illness among the Alaskan Eskimoes or the Aleuts of the Canadian Northwest Territories. *Look @ I touching => baby dies.*

10. Briefly explain what is meant by complimentary proteins.
amino acids – Lysine – methionine

11. Briefly give several examples of food restrictions often practiced by women in different cultures during the postpartum period.

5: Essay Questions

1. Explain how culture is learned, shared, adapts to particular environmental conditions, and   is dynamic. Provide an example in each case to support your explanation.

2. Using a particular culture with which you are familiar, identify a belief related to breastfeeding that is:
   a. beneficial
   b. harmless
   c. harmful
   d. uncertain

3. Explain the difference between viewing breastfeeding as an assumed way of feeding instead of as a method of feeding one is able to choose. Use at least two examples to support your distinctions.

4. Identify at least five different nonverbal messages that mothers receive regarding breastfeeding. You need not limit your answer to a single culture.

5. What is colostrum? Explain how it is viewed in different cultures and how these beliefs may influence how colostrum is used. Provide at least two examples to buttress your argument.

6. What is the "hot-cold" theory? On what is it based, and how does it influence food choices? Indicate how knowledge of this theory might be used when offering food to Hispanic women housed in a postpartum hospital ward?

7. What is the significance of green-tinged milk?

8. Offer at least three reasons for weaning. In each case, indicate in what culture(s) this belief is held.

6: Story Problem

You live in a large urban city. Among your clients are women who practice the following religions: Hinduism, Islam, Judaism, Catholicism, and Presbyterianism. Among your clients are a few women who are "vegan" vegetarians and several others who are "lacto-ovo-vegetarians." About 10% of your clients have their babies at home; the other 90% give birth in three of the five largest hospitals in the city. At a prenatal breastfeeding class, dietary restrictions are discussed.

1. How would you help all of the 20 women feel comfortable sharing information about the dietary restrictions they have practiced, or have been told they should practice?

2. Identify different restrictions which might be mentioned by one or more of your clients.

3. One of the class members asks you whether it is safe to fast, now that she is pregnant. What do you tell her?

4. Another class member tells you she "craves" foods that her religion does not allow her to eat. What do you tell her?

In the course of a home visit to a mother who gave birth 30 hours earlier, you notice that the woman's mother has prepared an aromatic drink which she wants to give to the baby as well as the new mother.

5. What do you do?

One of the mothers in your practice introduces you to her mother-in-law, who has recently arrived from Japan to help care for her daughter-in-law and the new baby. The grandmother intends to take care of the baby at night. The new father asks what he should tell his mother about bottle-feeding, since she insists that is how her "modern grandchild" should be fed at night.

6. What is your response?

7. Two weeks later, you receive a call from a mother who has been told that she should wean her baby <u>now</u>; she has nursed "too long." What does this mean? What do you suggest to the mother?

3

Birth = crisis ⇒ new ways of behav on family members

Families

1: Outline of the Chapter

Introduction
Family forms and functions
The effect of a baby on a family
Family theories
Fathers
    Attachment to the baby
    Breastfeeding
Levels of family functioning
    The teen-age mother
    The low-income family
    Obstacles to breastfeeding among low-income families
Social support systems
Breastfeeding promotion
    Breastfeeding programs that work
Summary

2: List of Key Concepts in the Chapter

The reader is urged to look for these key concepts in the body of the chapter and to develop questions deriving from these concepts as one way to gain understanding and insight into their relationship to lactation and breastfeeding. In this chapter, the reader may find it helpful to compare families representing different levels of functioning from different theoretical perspectives–noting how family form and function is related to likelihood of breastfeeding initiation and how different theoretical perspectives draw our attention to different elements within each family group.

Affiliation
Attachment
Contracting stage
Couple stage
Expanding stage
Extended family
Family development theory
Family of orientation
Family of procreation
Family functioning
Innovation-Decision Process
Nuclear family

3: Multiple-Choice Questions

1. When a second child joins a household consisting of a mother, father, and older sibling, how many relationships now exist between these four individuals?
    a. three
    b. four
    c. six
    d. ten

2. When a father has a new baby, he usually first touches the neonate with:
    a. his finger tips, as he strokes the baby's arm or leg
    b. his entire hand, as he holds the baby up for his wife to see
    c. his finger tips, as he strokes the baby's chest
    d. his face, when he offers a welcoming kiss

3. According to one investigator, a family in its own <u>adolescence</u>:
    a. is comprised of at least one teen-age parent
    b. needs a helper to point out the family's ability to cope
    c. has only one child
    d. all of the above

4. The Innovation-Decision Process attempts to explain why some low-income women choose to breastfeed and why others do not. Which of the following elements is the first step in innovative behavior?
    a. knowledge
    b. persuasion
    c. confirmation
    d. implementing the decision

4: Short-Answer Questions

1. Identify four elements considered universal to all families. Explain the importance of each element in understanding how a family functions.

2. Identify five different stages in the family life cycle. For each stage, identify when it is likely to occur, and at least one problem the family must deal with at that stage.

3. Many fathers assume that father-child closeness derives primarily from feeding. Briefly explain to a class of new fathers how narrowly this assumption frames the father's role. Give at least three examples of other ways in which a father can be close to his baby.

4. Offer an example of each of the following levels of family functioning. In each case, explain how breastfeeding might be encouraged as part of the health worker's plan of care for the family members.
   a. infancy
   b. childhood
   c. adolescence
   d. adult

5. Using each of the following characteristics, explain why a low-income family is unlikely to breastfeed:
   a. ethnic group
   b. lack of support
   c. lack of information
   d. hospital practices
   e. hospital-based formula marketing
   f. timing of solid-food introduction

6. Focusing on the same items mentioned in question #5 above, indicate how each can influence an affluent mother not to breastfeed.

5: Essay Questions

1. A baby represents many things to a family. Briefly discuss five different reasons for having a baby. In each case, note how each reason might influence a family member's behavior relating to other people, such as in-laws, friends, or colleagues.

2. Meet John. He has been a father for only three hours and has just arrived home from the hospital. On the way home, John was stopped by a policeman for

weaving all over the road. Only after explaining that he and his wife had just had their first baby, following a 12-hour labor, did the policeman send him home without giving him a ticket. John knows life will not be the same. Identify for him at least three aspects of "reality" that he needs to confront so that he can make his new parenting experience as positive as possible. At least one of these items should deal with breastfeeding.

3. Explain why many teen-age mothers prefer not to breastfeed.

4. Briefly discuss the importance of social support following a life stress. Use three different situations involving life stress–one of which is the birth of a new baby– to provide examples of the effect of social support on different family members.

5. What is an advocate? Using an outline of words or phrases, develop a breastfeeding promotion program that takes into account the following elements:
    a. the involvement of different family members
    b. the support of key community members
    c. the receptivity of people in power positions
    d. the resources available to those advocates for this breastfeeding promotion program

6. Explain how the following practices are related to effective breastfeeding promotion:
    a. attitude change on the part of health professionals
    b. rooming-in
    c. opportunity for early breastfeeding
    d. eliminating artificial feeding in the hospital

6: Story Problem

You have been hired to promote breastfeeding among the families served by a local clinic.

1. What do you need to know about these families before developing a program promoting breastfeeding?

You now know something about this clinic's population.

2. Describe it.

Taking into account the percentage of teen-age families, and the likelihood that some of them are composed of single women and their offspring, you present an interim plan to the clinic management.

3.   Outline your interim plan.

Several of the clinic staff "talk a good game," but your observations suggest that they do not really believe that breastfeeding is all that important. At least one is actively antagonistic and is waiting for you to fail.

4.   Define what that staff member means by "failure."

You believe that if the administration backs your efforts, you will be more likely to convince others on the clinic staff that your plan is appropriate and deserves to be implemented.

5.   How do you secure both the administration's active support and its financial backing?

You have set goals for yourself and for the clinic.

6.   Identify the current breastfeeding initiation and duration rates among the clinic's client population.

7.   Now tell us what your goals are for one, two and three years from now.

8.   How do you expect to reach those goals? Provide examples to support your answer.

SECTION

TWO

Anatomic and Biologic Imperatives

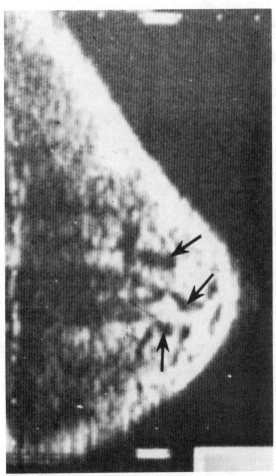

The breast. Arrows point out three milk ducts. (Thomas Jefferson University, Department of Radiology.)

4

Anatomy and Psychophysiology of Lactation

1 : Outline of the Chapter

The Mother
    Mammary development
    Structure
    Variations
    Pregnancy
    Hormonal influences during puerperium
    Lactogenesis and psychological influences
    Oxytocin
    Galactorrhea
Clinical implications
    Breast assessment
    Classification of nipple function
    Early frequent feedings
The infant
    Newborn oral development
    Suckling vs. sucking
    Breathing and suckling
Clinical implications
    Suckling assessment
Summary

2: List of Key Concepts in the Chapter

The reader is urged to look for these key concepts in the body of the chapter and to develop questions deriving from these concepts as one way to gain understanding and insight into their relationship to lactation and breastfeeding. In this chapter, the reader may find it helpful to consider those hormonal and other elements specific to the lactating mother–plus how assessment of breast and nipple tissue and infant anatomy can highlight specific management recommendations.

Breast assessment
Breast structure
Galactorrhea
Glucocorticoids
Hormones
Human placental lactogen (HPL)
Insulin
Lactogenesis
Mammary development
Newborn oral development
Nipple function
Oxytocin
Pregnancy
Prolactin
Prolactin inhibiting factor (PIF)
Suckling/sucking
Thyroid-stimulating hormone (TSH)
Thyrotropin-releasing hormone (TRH)

3: Multiple-Choice Questions

1. How does the tongue move with normal suckling at the breast?
    a. from back to front
    b. from front to back
    c. from side to side
    d. in an arrhythmic fashion so that the top of the areola is touched by the tongue throughout a feeding
    e. both b and c above

2. Following birth, what happens to serum prolactin when suckling occurs?
    a. it drops to baseline and remains there
    b. it peaks with each suckling episode, remaining at peak levels between feeds
    c. it peaks with each suckling episode, declining between feeds
    d. it gradually climbs over time

3. Scarring caused by burns to the breast and nipple:
    a. does not preclude breastfeeding
    b. may be an indication of more severe internal trauma
    c. nearly always means that the nipple pores have been destroyed
    d. b and c above

4.   Oxytocin secretion results in:
     a.   milk production
     b.   milk ejection
     c.   uterine contractions
     d.   all of the above
     e.   b and c above

4: Short-Answer Questions

1.   Briefly distinguish between suckling and sucking. During what time period does each occur?

2.   Describe how you would determine that a mother has retracted nipples. What is the difference between retracted and inverted nipples?

3.   What is suckling assessment and why is it important?

4.   What is meant by the phrase "obligate nose breather"? How is this related to infant feeding?

5.   Marked asymmetry of the breasts may indicate what?

6.   Distinguish between surgical procedures to the breast that are very likely, and less likely, to result in reduced milk production.

7.   What is galactorrhea?

5: Essay Questions

1.   Briefly discuss the notion that function changes as form changes in relation to breast size as a predictor of lactation success.

2.   Describe each of the following structures and distinguish between them as to where they might be found and their function in lactation:
     a.   lactiferous duct
     b.   adipose cells
     c.   milk glands
     d.   myoepithelial cells
     e.   nipple
     f.   areola

3. Explain the relationship between prolactin release, oxytocin release, milk production and milk ejection.

4. Distinguish between breastfeeding and bottle-feeding in terms of the following elements:
   a. sounds
   b. frequency of suckling
   c. breathing patterns
   d. mouth extension
   e. tongue placement and action
   f. lip flanging
   g. feeding duration

5. "What the baby does is a simple activity, involving negative pressure and swallowing what he obtains." Indicate whether you agree with this statement and, if so, why? If you disagree, how would you argue that this statement is simplistic and/or incorrect?

6. Explain what is meant by the "supply-demand" response.

6: Story Problem

You are asked to explain to a group of pregnant couples how the breast works.

1. Outline your presentation to this group.

One of the men asks," Now I know how the breast works, but the baby has to do something, too. Right?"

2. "Right," you say. What else do you tell the group?

The class includes two scientific types who act fascinated by the hormones of pregnancy and lactation.

3. In everyday language, explain the following and their respective roles in the lactation process:
   a. prolactin inhibiting factor
   b. thyrotropin-releasing hormone
   c. human placental lactogen
   d. thyroid-stimulating hormone

"But, if I decide not to breastfeed," says one young woman, "I really won't be hurting myself or my baby all that much, will I?"

4.   What is your response to her question?

Later that day, one of the class members calls you and asks if you can explain why she never made enough milk for her first baby. She would like to breastfeed again, but is unsure if it will be possible.

5.   What do you need to know about her last breastfeeding experience?

6.   Indicate what she tells you when you ask questions about her last breastfeeding experience.

7.   Armed with that information, what do you now tell her about her likelihood of successful lactation with her second baby?

5

The Biologic Specificity
of Breastmilk

1: Outline of the Chapter

Maturational changes
Energy, volume and growth
    Caloric density
    Milk volume
    Infant growth
Nutritional values
    Fat
    Lactose
    Protein
    Vitamins
    Minerals
    Renal solute load
Anti-infective properties
    Respiratory illness
    Otitis media
The immune system
    Cells
    Antibodies/immunoglobulins
    Non-antibody antibacterial protection
    Anti-inflammatory components
Bioactive components
    Enzymes
    Growth factors
    Hormones
    Taurine
Antiallergenic properties
Implications for clinical practice
Summary

2: List of Key Concepts in the Chapter

The reader is urged to look for these key concepts in the body of the chapter and to develop questions deriving from these concepts as one way to gain understanding and insight into their relationship to lactation and breastfeeding. In this chapter, the reader may find it helpful to consider those elements that are unique to human milk; that is, those not available in artificial baby milks or other foods given to neonates, as well as those elements that can be found in other foods. One issue to discuss is the bioavailability of those elements found in human milk. Are those elements also optimally available in other foods or fluids and what might their absence portend for short- and long-term nutritional health?

Antiallergenic properties
Antibacterial and antiviral protection
Anti-infective properties
Anti-inflammatory components
Composition of human milk
Epidermal growth factor
Hormones
Immunoglobulins
Infant growth
Milk volume
3: Multiple-Choice Questions

1. Human milk contains what percent of solids to support energy and growth?
    a. 10
    b. 20
    c. 35
    d. 50

2. In most studies of milk volume, what is the approximate total volume produced by most mothers after the first month of breastfeeding a single infant?
    a. 500 ml/day
    b. 800 ml/day
    c. 1000 ml/day
    d. this amount cannot be determined insofar as each mother's supply varies so markedly from other women at the same lactational stage

3. When observing infant growth patterns over time, what pattern can be said to characterize the breastfed infant?
    a. a very early accelerated rate of gain in the first three months, followed by a slower rate of growth for the next three months
    b. very slow rate of gain in the first three months, followed by a more rapid increase to age six months

    c.   a continuously slow but steady rate of gain through the first six months

    d.   no difference between breastfed and bottle-fed babies if the formula used is protein (soy)-based

4: Short-Answer Questions

1. When individuals refer to human milk as "white blood," to what are they referring?

2. Discuss each of the following factors in terms of its effect on milk composition and volume:
   a. the baby's expressed need for milk
   b. the mother's age
   c. the beginning of the feed
   d. the end of the feed
   e. the baby's gestational age
   f. the stage of mother's lactation

3. It has been reported that breastfed infants consume approximately 30,000 fewer kcal than bottle-fed infants by eight months of age. Of what significance to the individual baby is this finding? Of what significance to overall infant health is this finding?

4. Briefly discuss the role of human milk in reducing infant morbidity and mortality resulting from:
   a. diarrhea
   b. gastrointestinal infections
   c. upper respiratory infections

5. What is the "bifidus factor" and how does it protect the breastfeeding infant's gut?

6. What is the relationship between lactoferrin and iron? Explain why exogenous iron supplements might interfere with lactoferrin.

7. Briefly discuss allergy predisposition. Note when an infant is most likely to express such a reaction, the role of genetics in determining the likelihood of allergy expression, and the role of breastfeeding in reducing its likelihood of occurrence or severity.

5: Essay Questions

1. For each of the elements listed below, note both its primary role in nutritional integrity of the human infant and what can occur if the element in question is absent or present in less-than-expected amounts?
   a. fat
   b. fat-soluble vitamins
   c. iron
   d. protein
   e. water-soluble vitamins
   f. zinc

2. Briefly discuss the role of secretory IgA immunoglobulin, noting whether it is present in greater quantities in colostrum or in mature human milk. How is it thought to protect the newborn from pathogenic organisms?

3. Briefly describe the role of epidermal growth factor and its relationship to the development of the mucosal barrier.

4. Taurine has now been added to some bovine-based artificial baby milks. What role does it play in human growth and development? And why was it added to at least one brand of infant formula?

5. Outline a breastfeeding class presentation designed to inform your audience of expectant couples of the unique qualities of human milk and the ways in which this food is a superior nutritional and health-protective fluid when compared to the scientific formulations that can be purchased at the food store. Remember that your audience does not consist of analytical chemists, biochemistry majors, or graduate students in dietetics!

6: Story Problem

At the end of a three-week mini-course on human nutrition, you have been asked to present a 30-minute lecture about human milk to both first-year medical students and to students training to become physicians' assistants.

1. First, select three elements to call to the students' attention, recognizing that the PAs are interested in the clinical implications of what you have to say (that is, how they can use it when assisting the doctor to keep patients well), while the medical students are engrossed in learning "all the details of everything."

After your lecture, a student raises her hand and asks, "But, isn't it true that bottle-fed babies are more likely to grow better–that is, faster–than breastfed babies?"

2.   How do you answer this question, focusing on both the fat volume of human milk, and the total milk volume obtained in the first several months of life?

Another student stops you in the hall and asks if you will serve as a reviewer for his research project. He has decided to study iron levels in infants fed different formulas and compare them to the iron levels in infants who are breastfed.

3.   What studies should he review before proceeding?

4.   How might you help him with this research project?

5.   List at least five questions you need to ask him to verify that he can obtain the information he needs to answer his research question.

A week after your lecture, the course administrator for a graduate class in Human Nutrition asks if you will meet with 15 students in a seminar focusing on allergies. They want to know about the role of human milk in preventing or reducing the severity of allergic responses.

6.   Outline what you will say to this group of students, noting at least four different ways in which human milk can reduce the degree of severity of allergic responses or prevent the occurrence of allergy expression in infants.

After your presentation, several students begin talking at once. The loudest of the group challenges you: "Okay, so breastmilk reduces it. But what if my wife refuses to breastfeed? She thinks it's something only animals do!"

7.   How do you respond to this student and to his wife's alleged reaction to your earlier recommendation to breastfeed?

Another student asks, "I can see where breastfeeding would help, particularly in the face of a family history of allergies. But what if the woman has to go back to work? She won't be able to exclusively breastfeed then, will she?"

8.   How to do you respond to this concern, focusing on the distinction between exclusive and partial breastfeeding, rather than on why partial breastfeeding may occur? (Please do not refer to Chapter 15 to answer this question!)

6

Drugs and Breastfeeding

1: Outline of the Chapter

Passage of maternal drugs into breastfeeding infants
    Drug factors
    Maternal factors
    Infant factors
    Breast and milk factors
    Routes of transport
Drugs that affect milk volume
General information
    Analgesics, NSAIDSs and narcotics
    Anticoagulants
    Anticonvulsants
    Antihistamines
    Antimicrobials
    Antifungals
    Bronchodilators
    Cardiovascular drugs
    Diuretics
    Laxatives
    Neuropsychotropics
    Oral contraceptives
    Herbs
Clinical implications
Maternal addiction
Substance abuse
    Amphetamines
    Alcohol
Environmental contaminants
Clinical implications
Summary

2: List of Key Concepts in the Chapter

The reader is urged to look for these key concepts in the body of the chapter and to develop questions deriving from these concepts as one way to gain understanding and insight into their relationship to lactation and breastfeeding. In this chapter, the reader may find it helpful to consider three or more different classes of drugs. For each one, note its likely impact on the mother's symptoms, her milk supply, and the appearance of the drug in her milk, as well as its appearance (and in what concentrations) in the baby's serum. Additionally, for each drug considered, ask whether some other therapy can be used to alleviate the mother's symptoms –with less effect on her milk supply and/or on the baby's level of exposure to the drug in question.

Addiction
Drug diffusion
Environmental contaminants
Feeding frequency
"Guilty unless proven innocent"
Half-life
Infant age/maturity
Lipid soluble
Metabolism of a drug
Milk/plasma ratio
Molecular weight
"Phase distribution model"
Route of administration
Topical medications

3: Multiple-Choice Questions

1. Which of the following statement(s) is true?
   a. most drugs pass into human milk
   b. nearly all medications appear in moderate amounts in human milk
   c. most drugs are contraindicated in the breastfeeding mother
   d. b and c above
   e. all of the above

2. When is a drug taken by a mother most likely to negatively affect her fetus or infant:
   a. early in lactation, when the baby is less than one month old
   b. late in lactation, when the baby is suckling less frequently
   c. early in pregnancy, when the fetus is still developing
   d. late in pregnancy, when the baby is laying down fat stores

3. A mother is told to use fenugreek. Why?
    a. it is the least expensive item she can obtain at the drugstore
    b. it is known to dry up mother's milk without causing pain
    c. it is known to stop pain when applied to the skin
    d. it is an herb, known to be a powerful galactogogue

4. Which has the greatest effect on the infant's drug exposure from breastfeeding?
    a. the medication is easily obtained
    b. the medication is long-acting
    c. the drug has a short half-life
    d. the medication is lipid-soluble

4: Short-Answer Questions

1. Briefly discuss the implications of new, precise methods of measuring chemicals in maternal and infant serum and human milk.

2. Briefly discuss at least three different ways to minimize environmental contamination.

3. Identify at least six elements which can serve as guidelines when a breastfeeding mother must take a medication. In each case, indicate how each selected element reduces the likelihood of infant exposure to the drug.

4. Explain how the infant's age affects her or his reaction to a drug the baby's mother is taking.

5. What is the effect on an infant if the mother ingests alcohol? Distinguish between small, occasional drinks and chronic or frequent use.

6. Radioactivity is an environmental contamination having worldwide potential for serious side effects. In light of this, indicate what you would tell a mother who plans to visit the site of the Chernobyl explosion as part of a scientific investigative team. The mother has a three-month-old infant who is exclusively breastfed and who will go abroad with her, but who will remain outside the area under investigation.

5: Essay Questions

1.   Explain why your concern about the effects of a sleep medication used by the mother of a newborn within 18 hours after a cesarean birth might differ if the same mother, two months later, chooses to use the same sleep medication.

2.   Using the suggested questions in the boxed material entitled "Breastfeeding Mothers Needing Medications: Questions to Ask" as a start, role-play with a colleague who takes the mother's role. Note what other questions, if any, you might wish to ask when discussing the medication in question.

3.   Identify at least three sources for information about drug use during lactation. In each case, indicate whether you would, or would not, use the source when seeking information about drug use during lactation. Justify your answer.

6: Story Problem

A mother with a two-week-old baby asks you if she should continue to take her pain pills. Although she is feeling better each day, her cesarean incision site became infected; it has since begun to heal, but is still painful.

1.   What do you tell this mother? Explain your rationale.

A week later, this same mother calls you and says that her nipples are reddened and extremely painful. In the course of your discussion with her, you learn that she has been taking an antibiotic since her cesarean.

2.   What do you suspect may be the culprit? Why do you suspect this? What do you recommend?

Three weeks later, this mother calls to ask you if she can take the ephedrine her doctor has prescribed for her. Her asthma is back, and she needs to use her bronchodilator.

3.   What do you tell the mother? Explain your rationale.

Several months later, this same mother calls to tell you that she was digging in her garden, encountered the roots of poison ivy plants, and is swollen and itchy from contact with them. Her doctor gave her a shot of Benadryl, which made her very sleepy, and instructed her to use a lotion to control her itching. She is afraid to use it, fearing that the lotion on her chest area will harm the baby if he gets it into his mouth while breastfeeding. In addition, she is afraid that the lotion will be absorbed into her skin and hence into her milk with possible untoward effects. When she asked her doctor this question, he shrugged and suggested that she might want to wean "temporarily, or for good" now that her baby is seven months old.

4.   What do you say to her about her first concern? Her second concern?

5.   When she asks you if it is true that her baby really doesn't gain anything from breastfeeding anymore, how do you answer her?

7

Viruses in Human Milk

1: Outline of the Chapter

Human immunodeficiency virus
    Transmission
    Testing
    Course of disease
    Clinical implications
Herpes simplex
Chickenpox (Herpes zoster)
Cytomegalovirus
Rubella
Hepatitis B
Implications for practice
Summary

2: List of Key Concepts in the Chapter

The reader is urged to look for these key concepts in the body of the chapter and to develop questions deriving from these concepts as one way to gain understanding and insight into their relationship to lactation and breastfeeding. In this chapter, the reader is asked to consider the differences among the viruses discussed, as well as their common properties; knowledge of both will assist in making appropriate recommendations to clients and other health-care workers.

Chickenpox (Herpes zoster)
Cytomegalovirus
Hepatitis B
Herpes simplex

Human immunodeficiency virus (HIV)
Passive immunity
Retrovirus
Rubella
Seroconversion
TORCH
Viral transmission

3: Multiple-Choice Questions

1. Universal precautions designed to protect health workers against infection through contact   with patients apply to:
   a. semen
   b. vaginal secretions
   c. human milk
   d. all of the above
   e. a and b above

2. Electing a cesarean birth to avoid infecting the neonate is most often recommended when the woman has a history of which viral infection?
   a. herpes simplex
   b. toxoplasmosis
   c. rubella
   d. cytomegalovirus

3. Which of the following viruses is most prevalent in the adult population?
   a. herpes simplex
   b. hepatitis B
   c. cytomegalovirus
   d. rubella
   e. herpes zoster

4. Assuming the newborn receives passive immunity from the mother, about how long will this immunity last?
   a. about one week
   b. about one month
   c. about two months
   d. about three to six months

4: Short-Answer Questions

1. What is meant by the term intracellular?

2. What is an enveloped virus?

3. Under what circumstances might a mother with herpes zoster continue to breastfeed her infant?

4. Explain why rubella causes birth defects, but is not a cause for concern if it is found in human milk.

5. How might the incidence of Hepatitis B infection be reduced in neonates, according to one study reported in this chapter? How is breastfeeding related to neonatal infection rates?

6. "The concern of health providers should be directed at mothers who have an unidentified infection." What is meant by this statement? How is it related to the infant feeding method the mother has chosen?

7. Briefly explain the term "passive immunity."

8. Under what circumstances, for viruses other than HIV, should a mother not breastfeed?

5: Essay Questions

1. Develop a chart that includes the following headings: route(s) of transmission, the likelihood of infection in the neonate, whether the infection is acute or chronic, and means of preventing cross-contamination. Complete the chart by filling in information under every heading for each of the following viruses: HIV, herpes simplex, cytomegalovirus, herpes zoster, hepatitis B, and rubella. At the completion of your chart, what are the similarities among these viruses; in what way(s) do they differ?

2. Explain why the author of this chapter concludes that a viral infection in the mother is "rarely" a reason for terminating breastfeeding.

3. Develop a brief one-page statement designed to inform its readers of your views on the advisability of breastfeeding when the mother of a neonate has a viral infection. Include comments about the risk of breastfeeding an older child when the mother has a viral infection. Include examples relating to at least four different viruses in support of your policy statement.

6: Story Problem

You are asked to assist a mother who has expressed a desire to breastfeed. However, the herpes infection she has harbored since she was 20 years old became active shortly before she went into labor. Thus, she is now recovering from a cesarean birth, which was not how she had originally expected to give birth.

1.   What do you tell her about her illness?

2.   What do you tell her about the desirability of breastfeeding this baby?

As a precaution, this mother's baby must room-in with her throughout her entire hospital stay.

3.   What do you tell this mother in order to help her see how beneficial such 24-hour rooming-in will be?

Unlike the other babies being cared for on the unit, this neonate regains her birthweight before being discharged on day four with her mother. A nurse approaches you and asks if it is true that mothers with herpes "make more milk than normal."

4.   How do you answer this question?

A mother is housed in the room farthest from the newborn nursery. Her baby was stillborn, and the mother tested positive for HIV. You are asked to help this mother because she is complaining of breast engorgement.

5.   What kind of precautions do you take before entering her room? While helping her?

6.   How do you answer her implied question that her HIV status was what "killed my baby"?

A mother calls you two months after her baby's birth. She has contracted chickenpox, after having been exposed to the disease through her five-year-old child.

7.   What is your reply to her concerns about her breastfeeding baby's risk of contracting chickenpox?

SECTION

THREE

Prenatal and Perinatal Periods

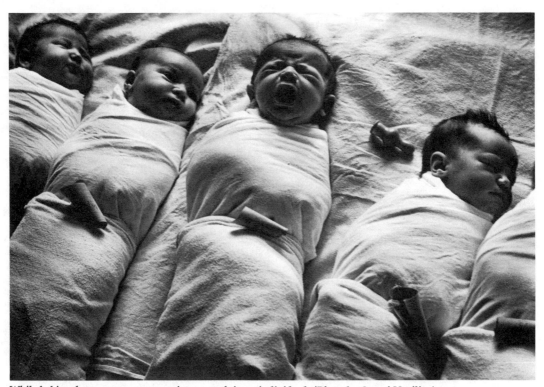

While babies share many common virtues, each is an individual. (Photo by Sergei Vasiliev)

8

Breastfeeding Education

1: Outline of the Chapter

Learning principles
Adult education
Teaching strategies
Parent education
Breastfeeding education for parents
    The infant feeding decision
    Practical information for early breastfeeding
    Continuing support for breastfeeding families
    Effectiveness of breastfeeding education
Methods and techniques
    Therapeutic communication
    Small group dynamics
    Educational materials
    Adapting education materials for special groups
    The team approach
Health-care provider education
    Staff education
    Continuing education
Curriculum development
    Developing learner objectives
The change process
A sample educational program
Summary

2: List of Key Concepts in the Chapter

The reader is urged to look for these key concepts in the body of the chapter and to develop questions deriving from these concepts as one way to gain understanding and insight into their relationship to lactation and breastfeeding. In this chapter, the reader is asked to consider the many ways in which expertise with lactation can be acquired, and the benefits and limitations of each option. In what ways do these options for professional lactation education mirror the educational resources for other health-care providers? Additionally, the reader may find it useful to evaluate local opportunities available to women for becoming informed about optimal infant feeding, and to see how such opportunities serve as an alternative to commercially advertised artificial feeding methods.

Adult education
Breastfeeding education
Change process
Continuing education
Curriculum development
Infant feeding decision
Learner objectives
Learning principles
Parent education
Practical information
Small group dynamics
Teaching strategies
Team approach
Therapeutic communication

3: Multiple-Choice Questions

1. Adult learners differ from children in which of the following ways:
    a. adults are self-directed
    b. time is considered the least valuable of all adult assets
    c. education must include the theoretical underpinnings of action
    d. all of the above
    e. b and c above

2. Which of the following purposes are common to most breastfeeding education programs?
    a. to support prenatal decision-making
    b. to provide practical information

    c.   to provide ongoing support
    d.   all of the above
    e.   a and b above

3.   For purposes of optimal learning, the ideal group size ranges from:
    a.   1-5 persons
    b.   3-7 persons
    c.   8-12 persons
    d.   13-18 persons
    e.   up to about 20 people

4.   The utilization model of curriculum development focuses on:
    a.   presenting information in the order of its usual occurrence
    b.   presenting information when participants most need it
    c.   moving from the simple to the complex when presenting information
    d.   moving from the known to the unknown when presenting information

4: Short-Answer Questions

1.   What is a "teachable moment"?

2.   Distinguish among auditory, kinesthetic and visual learning. How might breastfeeding skills be taught using each of these techniques?

3.   For each of the stages of acquisition to parenthood, identify two elements of learning new parents should master.

4.   Select at least five items about which breastfeeding mothers need information. Provide one or two sentences offering information about each item.

5.   What is therapeutic communication?

6.   Briefly identify at least three characteristics of effective educational materials.

7.   What is continuing education?

8.   Briefly explain how each of the following elements can limit the effectiveness of an educational program designed for health-care providers:
    a.   participants' lack of confidence
    b.   participants' sensitivity to failure
    c.   participants' poor self-concept
    d.   participants' resistance to change

9.   What is a change agent?

10. Briefly explain how a telephone "warmline" might be used to generate greater staff support for a more extensive program in breastfeeding education and support.

5: Essay Questions

1.   The authors suggest that breastfeeding education involves cognitive skills, affective learning, and psychomotor skills. Briefly identify elements of breastfeeding education   within each category and provide an example of each for both women wanting to learn how to breastfeed and health-care workers for whom knowledge of the lactation course is seen as appropriate to their area of specialization/practice.

2.   Select a specific topic pertaining to breastfeeding. Outline your teaching session, making clear its introduction, learning experience, and conclusion or summary.

3.   "Supplying information about breastfeeding management is sufficient to assure breastfeeding success." Debate the merits of this statement by providing at least two examples to support your contention that the statement is true and two examples of why the statement is false.

4.   Indicate how each of the following team members might contribute to a medical center's breastfeeding education program for health-care providers:
     a.   perinatal nurses
     b.   childbirth educators
     c.   dietitians
     d.   lactation consultants
     e.   community-based volunteer support groups
     f.   physicians

5.   Identify one aspect of a hospital or clinic setting that you wish to change as it relates to breastfeeding promotion, protection, or support. Outline how you would plan for that change, noting where resistance is most likely to come from and how you will counter such resistance.

6: Story Problem

You have been a member of the staff of a physicians' multi-specialty clinic for five years. In response to increasing complaints from patients about the lack of consistent breastfeeding information and support, you are asked to present a plan designed to improve the clinic's reputation as a "breastfeeding-friendly" care setting.

1. Why might you initially refuse the job?

2. What do you finally present to the medical staff? (An outline will do.)

3. Select two elements from your outline and add flesh to the bones of your proposal.

4. Explain where two forms of antagonism originate: one is overt, the other covert. Why have these reactions occurred and how do you plan to counter them?

5. Who among the staff are enthusiastic about your proposal? Why?

After several months of discussion, but little action, you meet with a group of other staff members to plan a strategy of "deliberative change."

6. Who among the staff are members of this group? Why have you selected them– or have you?

7. Outline your strategy of "deliberative change."

8. Indicate the reasoning behind your selection of the order of elements you have incorporated into your plan for change.

9. How do you plan to evaluate the effectiveness of your step-by-step plan? When do you plan to do such an evaluation? Why?

10. Where does patient education fit into your plan? Why there, rather than earlier or later?

9

The Breastfeeding Process

1: Outline of the Chapter

2: List of Key Concepts in the Chapter

The reader is urged to look for these key concepts in the body of the chapter and to develop questions deriving from these concepts as one way to gain understanding and insight into their relationship to lactation and breastfeeding. In this chapter, the reader is asked to evaluate policies and practices of a local hospital against the breastfeeding management recommendations offered. Note where current care patterns are appropriate practice and where practices need to be changed or protocols developed in order to incorporate newer practices into care plans.

Breast fullness
Breast refusal
Discharge planning
Engorgement
Feeding plan
Hypoglycemia
Insufficient milk supply
Leaking
Massage
Multiple infants
Sore nipples
Stooling
Suckling pattern

3: Multiple-Choice Questions

1. Rubbing the nipples and areola with a towel has been suggested as a way of preparing the nipple for breastfeeding. How do you respond to a question about doing so?
   a. It is unnecessary, and can make the mother more, rather than less, tender.
   b. It is appropriate if the mother is extremely gentle.
   c. It is appropriate if the mother succeeds in feeling a burning sensation; this means it is working.
   d. It is necessary only if the mother has very pale pink, or freckled, skin.

2. Following an unexpected cesarean birth, a mother may:
   a. feel that through breastfeeding she can prove herself as a mother
   b. feel that she has failed as a woman
   c. choose not to breastfeed for fear of failing again
   d. a and b above
   e. all of the above

3. When would transitory nipple soreness be most noticeable?
    a. between the first and second postpartum day
    b. between the third and the sixth postpartum day
    c. between the sixth and tenth postpartum day
    d. any time in the first two weeks, depending on the mother's complexion

4. Which of the following is likely to stimulate the mother to leak milk–particularly in the early weeks of breastfeeding?
    a. the scent of her baby's clothes
    b. thinking about her baby
    c. a crying baby
    d. b and c above
    e. all of the above

5. A problem of too much milk:
    a. almost never occurs in the developed world
    b. may occur when a baby receives an abundance of "foremilk," but is removed before receiving the later arriving "hindmilk"
    c. can be altered with a care plan that includes changes in certain aspects of her breastfeeding pattern
    d. b and c above
    e. all of the above

4: Short-Answer Questions

1. Identify at least three different ways in which a mother can prepare for breastfeeding.

2. Identify and briefly discuss at least five different fallacies or faulty assumptions pertaining to breastfeeding. Note why these assumptions are faulty and offer a more appropriate alternative explanation of the issue in question.

3. Identify three different ways of holding a baby for breastfeeding. In each case, specify when a mother might use each position and at least one caution pertaining to each.

4. What is hypoglycemia? Identify when it is most likely to occur in a neonate and explain the rationale regarding how the baby should be managed.

5. Answer each of the following questions with a sentence or two that characterizes a normal suckling pattern in the healthy newborn:

    a. What do the baby's cheeks look like?
    b. Where is the baby's tongue?
    c. What do you hear when the baby is suckling?
    d. How tight is the baby's seal on the breast?

6. Briefly explain what colic is, noting at least three different explanations for its occurrence in some babies.

7. Describe a feeding pattern often seen in neonates born in a hospital where rooming-in is practiced and mothers are discharged late on the second day or early on the third day postpartum.

8. Briefly distinguish between typical stooling patterns in an exclusively breastfed baby and a a baby receiving only artificial baby milk at the following time periods:
    a. Day 2
    b. Day 10
    c. Day 30
    d. Day 80

5: Essay Questions

1. Discuss at least four different reasons why early and frequent breastfeeding promotes optimal functioning in both mother and newborn. Show how each reason is related to the other reasons you have selected.

2. Distinguish between breast fullness and breast engorgement, noting when each is likely to occur. Briefly indicate how you would characterize each so that a mother could tell when they occur and would know what to do for herself following discharge from the birthing center as soon as 12 hours after the birth.

3. You are approached by a sales representative who is eager for your endorsement of a new nipple and breast cream which is soon to be released in the marketplace in all English-speaking countries. You note that the list of ingredients includes lanolin and a petroleum derivative. What is your reply to the sales representative? Justify your answer with at least three different reasons supporting your decision.

4. A mother comes to your office complaining that she thinks she doesn't have "enough milk" to feed her baby. Her baby is now 11 weeks old. The baby is in the 75th percentile for height and the 50th percentile for weight. Identify at least five factors relating to the baby and at least five other factors relating to the

mother which may have contributed to the mother's conclusion that she hasn't enough milk. For each factor, offer her a one- or two-sentence explanation designed to answer her concerns.

5.   What is discharge planning? Identify at least two areas of teaching that help the mother as she continues to breastfeed. Identify three signs that indicate the need for intervention.

6: Story Problem

You, as a lactation consultant, have recently joined a group of physicians–including one obstetrician, two family practitioners (one of whom practices obstetrics), one pediatrician, and one internal medicine specialist. One of the physicians is less informed about breastfeeding than her partners. One of your roles is to provide prenatal breastfeeding instruction to all pregnant families.

1.   Briefly outline the contents of your breastfeeding class, noting how you will respond to questions.

In addition to providing prenatal instruction, you are also expected to see all new mothers and babies during their hospital stay.

2.   Describe what you do in the hospital with these clients. How do you reply when one of the nurses on the postpartum unit asks <u>why</u> you ask the mothers to sit up in a chair, rather than lounge back in the bed, for early breastfeedings?

One of the mothers you saw in the hospital is breastfeeding without difficulty. Her roommate is faring less well. Her baby rarely stays on the breast more than one minute before appearing to fall asleep. By day three, the mother is severely engorged; her baby is jaundiced and bili-lights have been ordered for use at home after her discharge this afternoon.

3.   How do you assist this mother without increasing the other mother's anxiety? What do you tell the mother about reducing her engorgement and encouraging the baby to be more wakeful for feedings?

After the mother is discharged, you are unsuccessful in reaching her at home. A week later she calls you. Her baby is nursing better, and the engorgement is gone, but she was quite disappointed to learn from the doctor that her baby has not regained his birth weight. This particular physician feels that every full-term infant should have regained birth weight within seven days.

4. How do you respond to the mother's questions about having to use supplements without calling into question the doctor's comments to her?

10

Breastfeeding the Pre-term Infant

1: Outline of the Chapter

Phase One: Expression and collection of mothers' milk
    The decision to breastfeed
    Initial breastfeeding consultation
    Developing a milk expression schedule
    Securing a suitable breast pump
    Explaining NICU policies about bacteriologic surveillance of mothers' milk
    Storage of expressed mothers' milk
Phase Two: Gavage feeding of expressed mothers' milk
    Methods of gavage administration of EMM
    Adequacy of expressed mothers' milk and the use of human milk fortifiers
    Guidelines for administration
    Contaminants in expressed mothers' milk to be fed to pre-term infants
Phase Three: In-hospital breastfeeding management
    Scientific basis for early breastfeeding sessions
    Managing early breastfeeding sessions
Phase Four: Postdischarge consultation
    Scientific basis for postdischarge breastfeeding management
    Research-based protocols for the postdischarge period
Summary

2: List of Key Concepts in the Chapter

The reader is urged to look for these key concepts in the body of the chapter and to develop questions deriving from these concepts as one way to gain understanding and insight into their relationship to lactation and breastfeeding. In this chapter, the reader may find it helpful to discuss whether certain issues which are important when the infant is premature are also important when the infant is a healthy, full-term neonate. In some cases, insight into this concept can also be gained by comparing the period of hospitalization with the postdischarge breastfeeding period.

Bacteriologic surveillance
Breastfeeding management
Expressed mothers' milk
Expression schedule
Feedings from different containers
Gavage feeding
Human milk fortifiers
Test-weighings

3: Multiple-Choice Questions

1. When a mother's infant is admitted to the NICU, she is considered a breastfeeding "candidate":
   a. when she says she wants to breastfeed
   b. when she says she had planned to breastfeed
   c. when the baby is able to suckle the breast
   d. unless she indicates otherwise

2. Indecisive mothers will often choose to breastfeed a pre-term infant because:
   a. they really do want to breastfeed
   b. they recognize the health benefits of human milk for their baby
   c. they are trying to make up for the pregnancy that ended too soon
   d. a and c above
   e. all of the above

3. In most cases, the mother of a pre-term infant will find _____
   most effective in obtaining milk for her pre-term infant:
   a. hand expression
   b. a hand-operated breast pump
   c. an electric breast pump
   d. a battery-operated breast pump

4. The composition of human milk is such that it:
   a. meets the nutritional needs of the very low-birth-weight infant
   b. meets the nutritional needs of the low-birth-weight infant
   c. meets the nutritional needs of the healthy, full-term infant
   d. b and c above
   e. all of the above

4: Short-Answer Questions

1. Why should a milk expression schedule for the mother of a pre-term infant parallel the frequency with which a healthy, full-term newborn breastfeeds?

2. What protocols ensure that expressed breastmilk for the pre-term infant has minimal concentrations of bacteria?

3. Under what circumstances should a double-pumping collection kit be considered the standard of care?

4. Discuss each of the following barriers to in-hospital breastfeeding of the pre-term infant:
    a. not providing an adequate environment in which to breastfeed the infant
    b. requiring that the baby reach a certain weight or age before being allowed to breastfeed
    c. requiring that the baby bottle-feed successfully before being given an opportunity to breastfeed

5. Briefly explain why routine test-weighing is considered the standard of care for small pre-term infants.

6. Briefly discuss the following elements as indicators of readiness to breastfeed:
    a. coordination of suck-swallow-breathing
    b. gestational age
    c. infant weight
    d. apneic episodes during bottle-feeding and during sleep

7. Explain why each of the following infant responses should be monitored and the results documented during early breastfeeding sessions. In each case, identify how they can be monitored and indicate whether these are invasive or noninvasive.
    a. heart rate
    b. respiratory rate
    c. oxygen saturation or transcutaneous oxygen pressure ($TCPO_2$)
    d. body temperature
    e. test-weighing

8. What is cue-based feeding? Give two examples of different cues that can be used when evaluating the pre-term infant who has been breastfeeding for some time and has not yet been discharged from the hospital.

9. Briefly explain how you might answer a mother's questions about the appropriateness of continuing bottle-feedings after the baby has been discharged from the hospital.

5: Essay Questions

1. Identify three elements that should be included in an initial consultation with the mother of a pre-term infant, and briefly describe each.

2. Identify at least three factors that are barriers to frequent milk expression. Discuss how each barrier can be overcome when developing an action plan with the mother of a pre-term infant.

3. Briefly describe how expressed mothers' milk should be stored for later use.

4. The authors of this chapter note that there is an inverse relationship between infusion rate and lipid loss during gavage feedings. Why is this finding important? How might the effects of such a finding be minimized when caring for a pre-term infant?

5. Briefly describe and demonstrate two different optimal positions for breastfeeding the premature infant. Explain when each position might be used.

6: Story Problem

Georgia Townsend has just arrived on the postpartum floor. Her twin sons were born by emergency cesarean section at 28 weeks gestational age. Georgia saw both babies only briefly before they were whisked away to the NICU. You are the lactation consultant who works with mothers whose babies are in the NICU.

1. Describe your first conversation with Georgia.

Georgia's roommate has a healthy baby whose cry is lusty and frequent. Dorene is bottle-feeding her baby. When you see Georgia on her first wheelchair visit to the NICU, she tells you she is not sure she should breastfeed her babies, now named John, Jr., and Gilbert.

2. What is your response?

Georgia's husband, John, interrupts your conversation by insisting on showing her a piece of paper on which he has scribbled notes about what the doctor told him about their sons. One baby is on a respirator; the other needed such assistance for only the first 24 hours. He tells his wife that she <u>must</u> breastfeed because the doctor said the babies needed the milk. He looks to you for confirmation.

3.   What is your response to his implied question?

Three days after Georgia gives birth, her first baby dies. You learn about this in a tearful phone call late at night. She has not pumped her breasts since learning of the baby's death six hours earlier. She says she feels "flat."

4.   What do you suggest that she do between the time of the call and your first opportunity to see her later that day?

Georgia tells you that she still wants to give her milk to Gilbert. She asks if she will ever produce more than the 30cc that she is currently obtaining with the battery-operated breast pump she is using at home.

5.   What is your response?

Four weeks later, when Gilbert is 32 weeks adjusted gestational age, the doctor considers him stable and ready to try to breastfeed. Georgia has been looking forward to this day; now that it has arrived she holds back. Her eyes filling with tears, she asks, "What if he doesn't like me?"

6.   Now what do you do? Your reaction to the question, please.

To everyone's surprise and his mother's delight, little Gillie latches on to Georgia's left breast and suckles as if he has always been fed in this manner. He continues to suckle and swallow rhythmically in bursts, with longer pauses gradually predominating over 20 minutes. Then he falls into deep sleep.

7.   What do you tell the baby's NICU nurse after this first breastfeeding?

8.   What feeding plan do you then develop with Georgia and Gillie's primary nurse?

Three weeks after his first breastfeeding, Gilbert Townsend is discharged home. The pediatrician has asked Georgia and John to bring him to the office for a first visit in three days.

9.   What do you tell Georgia about:
      a.   using the electric breast pump that she has been renting?
      b.   breastfeeding Gillie?
      c.   John's questions about "making sure" the baby gets enough milk by giving him two extra bottles a day?

    d. signs that Gillie does not need anything but the breast?

    e. her fears that she will do "something wrong"?

    f. who will be available to answer her questions and hold her hand?

11

Pumps and Other Technologies

1: Outline of the Chapter

Concerns of mothers
Stimulating the milk-ejection reflex
Hormonal considerations
    Prolactin
    Oxytocin
Pumps
    Mechanical milk removal
    Evolution of pumps
Hand pumps
    Review of research
Battery-operated pumps
Electric pumps
Miscellaneous pumps
    Juice jar breast pump
    Ora'lac
    Venturi breast pump
Clinical implications regarding breast pumps
Sample guidelines for pump recommendations and pumping techniques
Common pumping problems
Nipple shields
    Review of literature
    Risks
    Responsibilities
    Weaning from a shield
Breast shells
    Recommendations for use

Feeding tube devices
    Description
    Situations for use
    Method of use
Clinical implications regarding feeding tube devices
    Other considerations
Summary

2: List of Key Concepts in the Chapter

The reader is urged to look for these key concepts in the body of the chapter and to develop questions deriving from these concepts as one way to gain understanding and insight into their relationship to lactation and breastfeeding. In this chapter, the reader may find it helpful to identify the array of breastfeeding technologies available to mothers in her community. Noting the problems these technologies have represented may assist the reader to use the information in the chapter to assess whether the technologies are appropriate or inappropriate and make recommendations that reduce the difficulties in using such devices.

Breast pumps
Breast shells
Feeding tube devices
Finger-feeding
Milk-ejection reflex
Nipple shields

3: Multiple-Choice Questions

1.   For optimal response to a breast pump, the milk-ejection reflex should be elicited:
    a.   before the mother begins pumping her breast
    b.   at the time the mother begins pumping her breast
    c.   after the mother has been pumping her breast at least two minutes
    d.   as long as milk begins to flow during the pumping session; when the milk-ejection reflex occurs is immaterial

2.   Which of the following devices is most often a source of milk contamination?
    a.   intermittent electric pumps
    b.   breast shells
    c.   feeding tube devices
    d.   battery-operated breast pumps

3. Which of the following instructions relate to the use of nipple shields?
    a. ask the mother to sign a consent form identifying the risks of using the device
    b. provide written instructions for temporary use of the device
    c. inform the primary care provider that the device is being used
    d. all of the above
    e. b and c above

4. Nearly all of the breastfeeding devices in existence today:
    a. are the products of a high-tech society
    b. reflect a societal predisposition to think of breastfeeding as difficult
    c. reflect earlier versions of devices invented hundreds of years ago
    d. signify the breastfeeding mother's need for assistance

4: Short-Answer Questions

1. Identify at least two alternatives to using a nipple shield. Explain why you would recommend each alternative.

2. What is the significance of the amount of pressure that can be generated by different breast pumps? What would you caution mothers regarding the generation of maximum pressure? Maintaining adequate pressure?

3. What is finger-feeding? When is it an appropriate alternative to bottle-feeding? Identify a major risk involving its use.

4. Briefly explain why nipple shields are sometimes referred to as a "quick-fix" approach to early breastfeeding problems. How is this approach related to their inappropriate use?

5. Briefly distinguish between different types of breast shells, noting at least one risk and benefit of each.

6. Identify two different problems women sometimes encounter when they use breast pumps. Briefly explain how you would assist a mother in overcoming these problems.

7. Briefly explain why there is no such thing as one pump that works for all women.

5: Essay Questions

1. Identify all of the different breastfeeding-related technologies available in your community. With which of these items have you had personal experience? Experience through a client's use of one or more of them? What problems have the devices been used to solve? What problems have the devices themselves posed?

2. Identify at least six different uses for a feeding tube device–three involving maternal situations and three involving infant situations. In each case, indicate how the feeding tube device can assist in feeding or resolve the problem presented.

3. Identify at least three problems that can occur with the use of breast shells. Distinguish between their use prenatally and in the postpartum period.

4. Identify six different characteristics of a breast pump, noting for each characteristic its importance for the breastfeeding mother.

6: Story Problem

Marie has called your office to ask for a consultation in advance of her baby's birth. She is interested in obtaining a breast pump, which she plans to use after delivery.

1. What information do you need to know before recommending a pump?

2. Under what circumstances would you recommend against using a breast pump?

Marie leaves your office without a pump; she has chosen to wait until after the baby is born before obtaining one. You see her a week later and learn that one nipple inverts with pressure, while the other one is everted. The baby prefers the everted one.

3. How do you help Marie?

4. Which device will you use, if any, to assist the baby in learning to take Marie's inverted nipple?

Marie's husband is skeptical about the use of any breastfeeding devices; he prefers to think of lactation as "natural."

5. How do you support his view while assisting Marie as she uses one or more devices?

6. Which devices has she chosen to use?

When Marie next has contact with you, it is because she thinks the baby has thrush. After seeing both of them you concur with her.

7. Why do you recommend that she use a breast shell during the period when her baby and her breasts are being treated?

A week later, a mother with a baby whose suck is extremely weak is referred to you by a physician.

8. How do you recommend that the mother get adequate amounts of milk into the baby?

9. What kind of milk do you recommend? Why?

10. If the mother is uncomfortable using a breast pump to increase her own supply, what do you recommend that she do?

11. What do you tell the baby's primary care-giver about your plans for this mother and baby?

This mother asks you how long you think it will take for her one-month-old baby to learn how to breastfeed correctly.

12. What is your reply? Explain the rationale behind your answer.

12

Jaundice and the Breastfeeding Baby

1: Outline of the Chapter

Early-onset (neonatal) jaundice
Pathologic jaundice
Factors associated with early-onset jaundice
    Infant characteristics
    Hospital routines
Routine therapy for early-onset jaundice
Late-onset jaundice
Clinical implications
Summary

2: List of Key Concepts in the Chapter

The reader is urged to look for these key concepts in the body of the chapter and to develop questions deriving from these concepts as one way to gain understanding and insight into their relationship to lactation and breastfeeding. In this chapter, the reader may find it helpful to consider how jaundice in the neonatal period is viewed in her community and to compare it to the presentation in this chapter. Where differences exist, one useful exercise would be to identify these differences and note when differences between current practice and suggested recommendations from this chapter can be reconciled with a minimum of disruption.

Conjugated bilirubin
Early-onset jaundice
Incipient vulnerable child syndrome
Late-onset jaundice
Nonhuman milk feeds

Pathologic jaundice
Serum bilirubin
"Starvation-induced" jaundice
Unconjugated bilirubin
Water supplementation

3: Multiple-Choice Questions

1. Which of the following characterizes late-onset jaundice?
    a. is present in 70% to 100% of all breastfed infants
    b. usually manifests itself in the second week of life or later
    c. in most cases requires no intervention
    d. b and c above
    e. all of the above

2. Which of the following characterizes early-onset jaundice?
    a. usually manifests itself 24 hours after birth
    b. in most cases requires no intervention
    c. can be influenced by the frequency and duration of nonmilk feeds
    d. a and c above
    e. all of the above

3. Which of the following reduces serum bilirubin levels in neonates?
    a. short, frequent feedings of glucose water
    b. frequent, unlimited breastfeedings
    c. breastfeeding approximately every 3-4 hours with supplements of glucose water between feeds as needed
    d. bili-light therapy from day two through day four

4. "Starvation-induced" jaundice can occur when:
    a. babies are fed infrequently at the breast
    b. babies are given water or glucose in place of milk feedings
    c. babies are fed infrequent bottle-feedings
    d. a and b above
    e. all of the above

4: Short-Answer Questions

1. Briefly describe the rationale behind each of the following questions as it relates to minimizing the likelihood of early-onset jaundice.

a.   How often is the infant put to breast?
b.   How is the baby suckling?
c.   What is the baby's stooling pattern?
d.   Besides breastmilk, what other fluids is the baby being given?
e.   When is the baby being breastfed during any 24-hour period?

2.   Briefly explain why Asian babies have higher serum bilirubin levels than Caucasian or black babies. What implications does this finding have for care relating to early-onset jaundice in Asian babies?

3.   A mother is asked to stop breastfeeding for two days in order for her jaundiced three-day-old baby to receive milk other than her own. The rationale for this request is not made clear to her. What would you tell her so that she understands the reasoning behind this request? Indicate why you consider this request appropriate or inappropriate in the overall care plan established for her baby.

4.   Briefly describe "incipient vulnerable child syndrome" and how a diagnosis of jaundice may contribute to it.

5.   What is pathologic jaundice? When is it likely to manifest itself?

5: Essay Questions

1.   Care of the jaundiced neonate often includes routines which have recently been questioned. Identify at least four such hospital routines and note at least two effects of those routines on the neonate which could contribute to an elevation in bilirubin. Also note whether and/or how these same routines could contribute to difficulty with breastfeeding.

2.   The authors of this chapter state: "It is appropriate...to examine those routines...which can be most easily altered or eliminated to reduce the likelihood that initiation of infant feeding *of any kind* in that institution contributes to early-onset jaundice." What do they mean by this statement?

3.   Briefly distinguish between early-onset jaundice and late-onset jaundice, noting at least four differences between them.

4.   Select at least four variables that have been found to influence the likelihood of the occurrence of "breastfeeding jaundice." Explain the significance of each of these variables to one another and to the likelihood of bilirubin elevation.

6: Story Problem

You receive a phone call from Monica Tremain. Her first baby was severely jaundiced and required bili-light therapy for several days before coming home. As a result, Monica stopped breastfeeding; she was convinced that her milk was the reason for the baby's yellow skin and lethargy. This mother is due to give birth to her second child in two weeks. She would like to breastfeed this baby, but she is fearful that her milk is "bad."

1.   What do you ask her about her experience with her first baby?

2.   What do you tell her to expect with this new baby?

Monica gives birth to a healthy boy, who shows an immediate interest in suckling for extended periods. After seeing colostrum dribble out of the baby's mouth, Monica exclaims, "Look how yellow that is! No wonder Gisèle was so yellow!"

3.   What is your response?

Gunter continues to suckle well throughout the hospital stay. On day three, the pediatrician reports to Monica that the baby's bilirubin level is 9. The doctor would prefer that it be lower and asks Monica to bring the baby in the next day for another blood sample. In the meantime, she is to supplement the baby with water after every feeding to "flush" the baby's system.

4.   How do you respond when Monica–convinced that her milk has again done something to her baby–tearfully relates this conversation to you? If your recommendation differs from the doctor's, how do you reconcile the two so that Monica continues to view her doctor as supportive of breastfeeding?

The next day, Monica learns that the baby's serum bilirubin has dropped to 3. She calls you triumphant; but she continues to harbor concerns because "the doctor told me it's now too low!"

5.   What do you tell Monica this time?

SECTION

FOUR

Postnatal Period

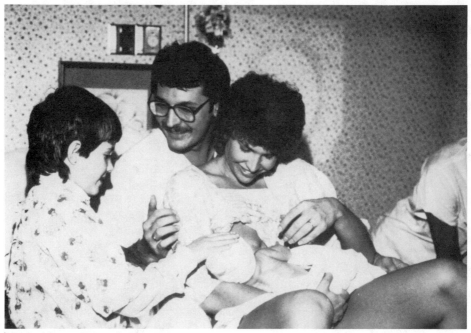

(Used with permission of Pat Bull.)

13

Maternal Health

1: Outline of the Chapter

Maternal nutrition: basic guidelines
    Foods that pass through milk
    Maternal weight
Alterations in endocrine and metabolic functioning
    Diabetes mellitus
    Thyroid disease
    Pituitary dysfunction
    Cystic fibrosis
Infections
Dysfunctional uterine bleeding
Relactation
Induced lactation
Impaired mobility
    Multiple sclerosis
    Rheumatoid arthritis
    Clinical implications
Seizure disorders
Postpartum depression
    Clinical implications
Asthma
Smoking
Diagnostic studies using radioisotopes
Discussion
Summary

2: List of Key Concepts in the Chapter

The reader is urged to look for these key concepts in the body of the chapter and to develop questions deriving from these concepts as one way to gain understanding and insight into their relationship to lactation and breastfeeding. In this chapter, the reader is asked to consider some of the implications of maternal illness on the lactation course and breastfeeding. Particularly helpful to the reader is a comparison between situations in which uneventful lactation is not an appropriate goal and those situations in which maternal illness need not contraindicate the lactation course.

Asthma
Cystic fibrosis
Diabetes
Dysfunctional uterine bleeding
Endocrine functioning
Hyperthyroidism
Hypothyroidism
Impaired mobility
Induced lactation
Infections
Maternal nutrition
Maternal smoking
Metabolic dysfunction
Multiple sclerosis
Pituitary dysfunction
Postpartum depression
Radioisotope studies
Relactation
Rheumatoid arthritis
Seizure disorder

3: Multiple-Choice Questions

1. Maternal nutrition has been found to have a _____ effect on the lactation course.
    a. significant (especially if the mother is undernourished)
    b. marginal (in most cases)
    c. significant (especially if the mother is ingesting a large quantity of fats)
    d. marginal (except when the mother is undernourished)

2. Insulin-dependent diabetes mellitus (IDDM):
    a. is an acute illness in the breastfeeding baby of the mother with diabetes
    b. is a chronic illness in the mother; she should be discouraged from breastfeeding
    c. is a chronic illness in the mother; she should be encouraged to breastfeed
    d. a and b above

3. Which of the following maternal conditions is likely to be reflected in poor weight gain in the baby?
    a. hypothyroidism
    b. hyperthryoidism
    c. diabetes mellitus
    d. prolactinoma

4. When a woman has cystic fibrosis she:
    a. should be strongly discouraged from breastfeeding in order to protect her own health
    b. will produce milk that is insufficient to meet her baby's needs
    c. needs close nutritional monitoring to maintain her own health
    d. should not breastfeed because of the bacterial pathogens she carries

5. Which of the following conditions precludes breastfeeding?
    a. rheumatoid arthritis
    b. any generalized seizure disorder
    c. postpartum depression
    d. all of the above
    e. none of the above

4: Short-Answer Questions

1. What is the difference between an acute and a chronic illness? Select one example of each.

2. Briefly discuss the relationship between weight loss and maternal exercise during lactation.

3. What is a prolactinoma? How does it influence lactation?

4. What is a "self-limiting" illness? Briefly explain how antibiotic therapy for such an illness will affect the breastfeeding baby of a mother receiving such therapy.

5. Explain how excessive bleeding in the postpartum period can negatively affect the lactation course.

6.   Briefly explain why one cannot predict whether/when an adoptive breastfeeding mother will develop a milk supply sufficient to completely nourish the breastfeeding baby. Refer to at least one maternal and one infant factor in your answer.

7.   What is multiple sclerosis? How does it affect the mother choosing to breastfeed? Her breastfeeding baby?

8.   Briefly explain how a mother might avoid exposing her baby to radioactive isotopes following a diagnostic study requiring their use.

9.   Briefly outline what foods you would encourage a breastfeeding mother to eat and which she should avoid if she is concerned about losing excess weight she gained before she became pregnant and maintaining sufficient energy to make "good" milk for her baby.

10.   Briefly discuss at least five recommendations you would make to a mother with limited   mobility. In each case, indicate your reason for offering such a recommendation.

5: Essay Questions

1.   A mother with a history of epilepsy asks how she might make her home safe for her baby in the event she has a seizure. What do you suggest to her? Why?

2.   For each of the following, indicate the effect on either the lactation course or the breastfeeding infant:
     a.   calcium
     b.   vitamin D
     c.   folic acid
     d.   the age of the mother
     e.   fatty acids
     f.   vitamin B_6
     g.   iron
     h.   caffeine

3.   Distinguish between relactation and induced lactation. Identify at least two benefits of these lactation options and two potentially negative consequences.

4.   From a hormonal perspective, what is the normal postpartum state? How does this relate to postpartum depression? To usual treatment regimens? To the mother's plan to breastfeed?

5. Indicate how nicotine addiction influences milk production and the breastfeeding infant. What is the most appropriate recommendation to make to a nicotine-addicted mother regarding breastfeeding prior to her baby's birth?

6: Story Problem

You are part of a private practice only recently affiliated with a major medical center. You have been asked to speak to a group of residents in internal medicine about breastfeeding in the event of maternal illness.

1. Outline that portion of your talk which focuses the residents' attention on the normal course of lactation for the healthy mother.

2. Distinguish among the healthy, the acutely ill, and the chronically ill mother who wishes to breastfeed. Justify the distinctions you have made and those elements that need not be different for the mother with an illness.

In the midst of your presentation, a hand is raised in the back of the room. Your host has warned you in advance of your presentation that the chairman of the department is from "the old school." She doesn't believe that breastfeeding is safe if the mother is on any kind of drug. You suspect that the distinguished-looking older woman waving her hand is the chairman. She asks, "What about the mother taking medications?"

3. Outline your answer, making sure that you include a response that includes medications used to treat an acute illness, a chronic illness, postpartum depression, and following a radioisotope scan. NOTE: The choice of illness in each case is yours!

The same hand waves again. "It sounds to me like you are saying.... Is that right?"

4. Tell us what the physician has said to you. How do you make her interpretation of your comments more accurate ?

Your lecture is over. Several residents approach you during the break between lectures. One tells you his sister is adopting a baby and wants to breastfeed. He wants some advice he can give her when he sees her over the New Year holidays.

5. What do you ask him before replying to his question?

6. What information do you offer that he can take home to his sister?

Another resident calls you at your office a few days after the lecture. She has a breastfeeding patient whom she has treated for asthma. She now suspects that this patient has returned to smoking, a behavior that the resident had strongly discouraged. The patient is worried about her baby's behavior, which includes colic. The pediatrician has offered "relaxing drops" for the baby, which the mother is not comfortable with. The resident wants to know if it is possible for the baby to be reacting to the mother's smoking.

7.   How do you respond?

The chairman of the Department of Internal Medicine calls to thank you for "a most interesting presentation last month." She asks if you will make another presentation–this time to the entire faculty.

8.   How do you respond to her compliment and request?

She then tells you that she would prefer that you "downpedal" your notion that nearly all women can and should breastfeed because the department's grand rounds presentations are followed by a dinner which is paid for by one of the pharmaceutical companies that manufactures artificial baby milk. "After all, we don't want to lose the good will we've developed with them. They might not want to pay for our dinners," she laughs.

9.   How do you reply to the chairman's request regarding what you are to say?

14

Breast-Related Problems

1: Outline of the Chapter

> Nipple variations
> > Inverted or flat nipples
> > Large/elongated nipples
>
> Plugged ducts
> Mastitis
> Skin rashes and lesions
> > Candidiasis/thrush
>
> Breast pain
> Milk blister
> Mammaplasty
> > Breast reduction
> > Mastopexy
> > Augmentation
>
> Breast lumps and surgery
> Fibrocystic disease
> Bleeding from the breast
> Breast cancer
> > Effect of radiation and chemotherapy
>
> Clinical implications
> > Mastitis
> > Breast surgery and abscess
>
> Summary

2: List of Key Concepts in the Chapter

The reader is urged to look for these key concepts in the body of the chapter and to develop questions deriving from these concepts as one way to gain understanding and insight into their relationship to lactation and breastfeeding. In this chapter, the reader is asked to consider how a variety of breast-related problems may influence the lactation course for the mother and her breastfeeding baby. Some of these problems will occur with relatively high frequency; others are considerably less likely. In all cases, however, the health of the mother and baby must be foremost when making recommendations.

Breast augmentation
Breast cancer
Breast reduction
Candidiasis
Fibrocystic breast disease
Intraductal papilloma
Inverted nipples
Mastitis
Mastopexy
Nursing diagnosis
Plugged duct
Prolactinomas

3: Multiple-Choice Questions

1. Which of the following is most likely to be associated with mastitis?
    a. plugged duct
    b. cracked nipple
    c. fatigue
    d. stasis

2. Prolactinomas:
    a. are pituitary tumors
    b. are a contraindication to breastfeeding
    c. tend to grow wildly during lactation
    d. b and c above
    e. all of the above

3. Women with a history of treatment for breast cancer:
    a. should not consider breastfeeding
    b. are unable to breastfeed after the surgery and/or chemotherapy
    c. represent many unanswered questions for the medical community
    d. a and b above
    e. none of the above

4. If the mother has an inverted nipple:
    a. the nursing baby is seldom precluded from suckling and obtaining milk
    b. the breast does not function well; thus, lactation should not be attempted
    c. the breast produces milk, but the nipple does not function sufficiently to sustain the infant
    d. breastfeeding proceeds more easily with the first baby than with later ones, for whom the inversion becomes more severe

4: Short-Answer Questions

1. Briefly discuss at least five recommendations for the treatment of a plugged duct.

2. Briefly discuss breast reduction surgery, noting when it is <u>most</u> likely to interfere with breastfeeding.

3. What is mastopexy and how is it done? Note whether it affects a woman's subsequent lactation course.

4. Briefly describe fibrocystic breast disease. How does it affect breastfeeding?

5. What is an intraductal papilloma? How is it identified and what is its effect on subsequent lactation?

6. Briefly distinguish between infectious and noninfectious mastitis. In what ways would the treatment for the two differ?

7. What is a "bleb"?

8. Briefly define a nursing diagnosis and indicate how it might be used to assist the lactation consultant in clinical practice.

5: Essay Questions

1. What is the difference between breast augmentation and breast reduction surgery. In your discussion, distinguish between the two in terms of:
    a. the woman's reaction to subsequent difficulty with breastfeeding
    b. the likelihood of difficulty with breastfeeding
    c. the nature of the surgery itself

2. Discuss at least four factors that can contribute to development of mastitis. Indicate how each factor is related to the others and what you would recommend to assist the mother in resolution of the problem.

3. How do you identify candidiasis/thrush in the baby's mouth? On the mother's breasts? In both cases, what is an appropriate remedy?

6: Story Problem

You feel assaulted by problems. In the past 10 days, you have fielded questions and seen mothers with the following concerns: recurrent plugged ducts; mastitis; four cases of thrush; a breast abscess; one woman who wants to breastfeed following augmentation surgery; and, three women who have had breast reduction surgery.

1. What do all of these women have in common?

2. Which of these women is least likely to be able to breastfeed completely?

3. Whom among this group have you asked to stop breastfeeding for two days in order to protect the baby?

4. In what sense do the mothers who have had surgery represent a problem of postindustrial society?

5. Following your visits with the women who have had reduction or augmentation surgery, what would you like for their cosmetic surgeons to know before they perform the same surgery on another woman in her childbearing years?

The woman with the recurrent plugged ducts asks you if her diet may have anything to do with her problems.

6. What is your reply?

She then asks what else she could be doing "wrong" that might be contributing to her difficulties.

7. After observing her baby at the breast, what is your answer to her question?

The phone rings; it is one of the clients with whom you worked for many weeks to clear up numerous early difficulties. She is tearful and confides: "I've found a lump in my breast–near my armpit. I'm scared to death. My mother died of breast cancer when I was 12. What should I do?"

8. Tell us your answer.

15

Maternal Employment and Breastfeeding

1: Outline of the Chapter

Why women work
Prenatal planning/preparation
The puerperium
Returning to work
    Breast pumping/expressing
    Storage
At work and at home
    Feeding options
    Loss of sleep
    The triple breeder-feeder-producer
Maternity leave
The "war" between work and home
The importance of social support
    Health-care workers: a special case?
The day-care dilemma
Clinical implications
Summary

2: List of Key Concepts in the Chapter

The reader is urged to look for these key concepts in the body of the chapter and to develop questions deriving from these concepts as one way to gain understanding and insight into their relationship to lactation and breastfeeding. In this chapter, the reader is asked to consider how paid employment outside the home alters women's plans for themselves and their babies and how those plans can continue to include breastfeeding. In some cases, comparing the at-home mother with her neighbor who leaves for work each morning might highlight specific clinical concerns designed to assist the employed breastfeeding mother.

Bottle-feeding
Breast pumping
Cup-feeding
Day-care
Expressing milk
Fatigue
Maternity leave
Milk storage
Prenatal planning
"Reverse cycle nursing"
Social support
Spoon-feeding
The "5-15-5" rule

3: Multiple-Choice Questions

1. For which of the following reasons do mothers express milk when they are regularly separated from their babies?
   a. to remain physically comfortable on the job
   b. to reduce the likelihood of leaking while on the job
   c. to collect milk for later use by the baby
   d. a and b above
   e. all of the above

2. "Reverse cycle nursing" refers to:
   a. altering the cycling pattern of a breast pump in order to increase the pressure it exerts on the breast
   b. the baby who sleeps more in the mother's absence and is more wakeful when she is available
   c. the mother who changes her pattern of breastfeeding at home to mimic that which occurs when she is at work

3. Job-sharing refers to:
   a. what a husband does when he works at home full-time and his wife works outside the home full-time
   b. when two individuals work part-time in the same position, as opposed to one employee who works full-time in the same position
   c. what happens when an employee does part of her work at home and part of her work at home

4. Spoon-feeding is possible:
   a. once the baby is able to sit up unaided
   b. when the baby can be safely propped into a highchair
   c. when the baby is at least two months old

  d.   from birth onward
  e.   after cup-feeding has been mastered

4: Short-Answer Questions

1.   Briefly distinguish between different day-care settings, noting the positive and negative aspects of each setting.

2.   Briefly offer at least three recommendations the employed mother may wish to consider when she plans to store her expressed milk for later use.

3.   Identify at least four questions a mother should ask if she is planning to use a breast pump.

4.   Identify at least three illnesses which are apt to occur when an infant or young child is cared for outside her/his own home. In each case, note whether breastfeeding is likely to reduce its incidence or severity.

5.   Identify five different individuals who can serve as a source of social support for the employed breastfeeding mother. In each case, provide an example of what they can do to help the person they are serving.

6.   Explain the difference between the length of a breast pumping experience and the duration of specific pumping sessions when seeking to obtain optimal breastmilk for later feedings. How would you recommend that a mother express or pump her milk in order to obtain as much milk as possible?

7.   Explain the "5-15-5" rule and how it relates to maintaining physical comfort on the job.

8.   When is the mother most likely to experience each of the following, and what would you recommend to her in order to avoid or reduce each item's effect on her upon her return to work?
  a.   engorgement and/or leaking
  b.   the baby's frequent changes of feeding patterns
  c.   concern about an inadequate or fluctuating milk supply
  d.   the need to express or pump milk

5: Essay Questions

1.   Using three of the four case studies at the end of Chapter 15, answer the accompanying questions, noting the different considerations among the cases,

as well as their similarities. Upon completion of the three cases, summarize key concerns most likely to affect breastfeeding duration when a woman goes to work or school shortly after the birth of her baby.

2. Using the following issues, explain to a colleague how you will assist a breastfeeding mother who has returned to work and does <u>not</u> want to use any artificial baby milk. Compare your recommendation in that situation to one in which the mother does not plan to express her milk, even when she is at home. In each case, touch on the five elements listed below:

   a. When will she return to work?
   b. How long will she breastfeed?
   c. Will she express or pump milk?
   d. Will she give her baby artificial baby milk for missed feedings?
   e. Where will the baby be cared for?

3. Identify at least four barriers to breastfeeding after returning to paid employment. In each case, indicate how each barrier can be reduced or eliminated so that it no longer serves as a reason for not breastfeeding.

4. Briefly discuss the issues involved in the timing of a breastfeeding woman's return to work–including her total work hours/week and projected breastfeeding duration. What would you recommend to an employed breastfeeding mother who wishes to continue breastfeeding longer than six months?

6: Story Problem

Joan Williams is planning to return to work after her baby's birth. She has asked for a prenatal consultation to make plans so that her baby's presence will not interfere with her career plans.

1. How do you respond to her questions?

One of your colleagues overhears Joan's questions and quips, "Good luck! There's no baby alive who's ever taken into account his mother's career plans!" Joan bursts into tears.

2. What do you say to Joan? Your colleague?

Joan's baby is born following a 35-hour labor which culminates in an assisted vaginal birth, resulting in moderate to severe blood loss and severe tearing of the perineum. At three weeks postpartum, Joan is still complaining about her hemorrhoid pain, tiredness, and nipple tenderness. Her baby cries a great deal, and Joan is tired of taking the additional iron pills which her doctor has prescribed. She plans to return to work next week and wants your advice.

3.   What do you tell her?

Joan calls you from the office two days after returning to work. She is crying. "What am I going to do?" she sobs. "I can barely walk, much less run up and down stairs all day. I went into a big meeting and leaked all over the front of my blouse when one of my bosses asked about the baby. And Jason kept me up all last night wanting to nurse. Everytime I tried to put him down, he cried and fussed.I'm exhausted—and it's only 2 o'clock! I have to be here for at least another three hours!"

4.   What is your reply?

Joan calls in sick the next two days and goes to bed with the baby. She forgets to take the iron pills and finds that she is less gassy and the baby is less fussy. "Is there a connection there?" she asks.

5.   How do you reply? What explanation do you give her?

Two months later, Joan calls you asking for referral for a new baby sitter. She is unhappy with the current sitter; her husband thinks she is simply unhappy having to leave the baby for 10 hours a day. She reports having asked the sitter to use a cup rather than a bottle to feed the baby. The sitter contends that the baby will choke and she will not be responsible!

6.   What is your response?

16

Fertility, Sexuality and Contraception during Lactation

1: Outline of the Chapter

Fertility
    The demographic impact of breastfeeding
    Mechanisms of action
    Lactational amenorrhea
    Silent ovulation
    The suckling stimulus
    Supplemental feeding
    The repetitive nature of the recovery of fertility
    The Bellagio consensus
Sexuality
    Libido
    Sexual behavior during lactation
Contraception
    Timing the commencement of a family-planning method: The double-protection dilemma
    The contraceptive methods
Clinical implications
Summary

2: List of Key Concepts in the Chapter

The reader is urged to look for these key concepts in the body of the chapter and to develop questions deriving from these concepts as one way to gain understanding and insight into their relationship to lactation and breastfeeding. In this chapter in particular, the reader is cautioned to consider each concept from at least two perspectives: both in the absence of lactation and during lactation. In some cases, insight into the concept can also be gained by comparing the prepregnancy period with the postbirth period.

Amenorrhea
Contraception
Double protection
Family planning
Fertility
Intercourse
Libido
Ovulation patterns
Sexuality
Supplemental feeding

3: Multiple-Choice Questions

1. When a mother breastfeeds at least seven times daily, ovulation is prevented from occurring.
    a. True: In exclusively breastfeeding mothers the frequency of suckling prevents ovulation.
    b. False: Even in exclusively breastfeeding mothers the frequency of suckling does not prevent ovulation.
    c. True: Ovulation is especially unlikely in the second six months of the child's life when frequent suckling occurs.
    d. False: Only in nutritionally at-risk mothers will frequent suckling stimulation inhibit ovulation.

2. The Bellagio consensus contends that:
    a. breastfeeding provides more than 75% protection against pregnancy during the second six months postpartum
    b. breastfeeding provides more than 75% protection against pregnancy during the first six months postpartum
    c. breastfeeding provides more than 98% protection against pregnancy during the first six months postpartum
    d. breastfeeding provides less than 15% protection against pregnancy during the second six months postpartum

3. In many developed countries, frequency of sexual intercourse _____ following the birth of a baby.
    a. declines over time
    b. increases over time
    c. declines and then increases
    d. increases and then declines

4. Which of the following delays first ovulation and subsequent risk of pregnancy?
    a. frequency of infant suckling
    b. daily duration of infant suckling
    c. supplementation of the infant's diet with nonhuman milk foods/fluids
    d. a and b above
    e. all of the above

4: Short-Answer Questions

1. Identify at least one permanent and one nonpermanent method of nonhormonal contraception–and two methods of hormonal contraception.

2. What is the Lactational Amenorrhea Method (LAM) of contraception?

3. What is "silent ovulation," and how might one suspect that it has occurred during lactation?

4. Briefly explain the effect of suckling stimulus on:
    a. the maintenance of milk production
    b. inhibition of ovulation
    c. milk ejection

5. When is the so-called period of "double protection" likely to occur?

6. Distinguish between pregnancy prevention and child spacing.

7. Briefly explain the role of the following in the normal menstrual course of a nonlactating woman:
    a. GnRH
    b. luteinizing hormone (LH)

8. How are levels of LH changed in a lactating woman compared to a woman who is not producing milk for a suckling infant?

5: Essay Questions

1. What is the relationship between contraception, fertility, sexuality, and lactation?

2.   Discuss the risks and benefits of at least five different contraceptive methods during the lactation course. In each case, identify at least one risk and one benefit to the lactating mother and/or her breastfeeding infant when such a method of contraception is used.

3.   Identify which method of contraception you would recommend in each of the following situations. Justify your answer in each case.
     a.   A woman of color, age 15, who has never used contraception in the past and who gave birth to an infant who died yesterday, 22 days after birth.
     b.   A woman with two living children, ages 13 months and 2 weeks, respectively. She is married and her husband strenuously objects to using condoms.
     c.   A woman with a newborn infant who is currently breastfeeding 12 or more times daily. This mother previously used an oral contraceptive, but is hesitant to do so while she is lactating.
     d.   A woman with a one-month-old infant. Her religious affiliation precludes limiting the number of children born to her and her mate. While she is fearful that her children will be born "too close" together, she is reluctant to use a method of contraception that is "obvious."
     e.   A mother with her fifth child, the last two of whom are only 15 months apart. The mother has breastfed all her children and intends to do so with her new baby as well. She fears having another pregnancy because of financial problems and concerns about how she will house and clothe her family.

6: Story Problem

Yolanda is 22 years old; she had her first child six weeks ago. Manuel, the father of her baby, is thrilled to be a new father and has already expressed his desire for more children. Yolanda is breastfeeding and wants more children–"but not right away."

1.   How do you address Yolanda's partner's desire for more children while supporting Yolanda's wish not to get pregnant quickly?

2.   What methods of birth control/child spacing would you discuss with these new parents? Why would you choose these methods to discuss?

In the course of your discussion, you learn that Yolanda's partner has been pressuring her to have intercourse. However, the first time they did so after the baby's birth, Yolanda experienced a great deal of pain. She offered to help him have an orgasm but refused to allow him to penetrate her vagina.

3.   What would you tell them about intercourse in the early postpartum period?

4. How would you counter Manuel's conclusion that Yolanda's breastfeeding is making intercourse painful for her?

Yolanda wants to use condoms and a spermicidal foam/jelly; Manuel does not. He prefers that Yolanda go on the pill if she <u>must</u> protect against pregnancy until their baby is a bit older.

5. How would you help them to see which of these choices may be appropriate for Yolanda while she is breastfeeding?

6. What other factors would you raise as they consider the risks and benefits of these methods of contraception?

7. Sexual feelings in the postpartum period reflect many aspects of parenthood. What information should you share with Yolanda about her own psyche and body responses–and those of her partner–in order to help her understand why their responsiveness may differ from their sexual expression prior to parenthood?

Manuel wants Yolanda to stop breastfeeding. He does not trust that she will not become pregnant–even when they are using "something else."

8. What do you need to know about Yolanda's lactation course and the baby's breastfeeding behavior in order to assess how likely Yolanda is to become pregnant:
    a. when her baby is less than three months old?
    b. when her baby is between four and six months old?
    c. when her baby is more than six months old?

17

Child Health

1: Outline of the Chapter

Growth and development
    Physical growth
    Weight and length
    Senses
    Reflexes
    Levels of arousal
Theories of development
    Nature vs. nurture
    Erikson's psychosocial theory
    Piaget's cognitive theory
Social development
    Language/communication
    Attachment/bonding
    Temperament
    Stranger distress
    Separation
Implications for practice
Immunizations
Dental health
Solid foods
    When should they be introduced?
    When should they be offered?
    Where should solid foods be given?
    Why should solids be delayed?
Obesity
Weaning
Implications for practice
Summary

2: List of Key Concepts in the Chapter

The reader is urged to look for these key concepts in the body of the chapter and to develop questions deriving from these concepts as one way to gain understanding and insight into their relationship to lactation and breastfeeding. The reader is asked to pay particular attention to normal growth and development and to how the experience of breastfeeding relates to such growth.

Arousal
Attachment
Communication
Dental health
Habituation
Immunization
Nature vs. nurture
Obesity
Reflexes
Senses
Separation
Social development
Stranger distress
Temperament
Weaning

3: Multiple-Choice Questions

1. How might a mother respond to the crying of a six-to-twelve-month-old child?
    a. provide lots of cuddling and holding
    b. offer foods easily handled by the child himself
    c. make sure the baby is the first in his age group to begin a certain food
    d. all of the above
    e. a and b above

2. Weaning which occurs rapidly may require that the mother:
    a. express or pump her breasts to reduce fullness
    b. avoid holding the baby lest he ask to nurse
    c. use cold showers to reduce the likelihood of breast leakage
    d. b and c above

3. Dental caries in breastfed children are caused by:
    a. suckling the breast through the night
    b. eating solid foods containing large amounts of sugar
    c. using a pacifier that is coated with sweeteners

    d. b and c above
    e. all of the above

4. Immunization of breastfed children:
    a. should be delayed until after weaning from the breast to assure that the immunization "took"
    b. usually results in a higher antibody level than in artificially fed children
    c. should be repeated after weaning to verify that the immunization "took"
    d. a and c above

5. In the first year a baby's:
    a. weight usually doubles
    b. weight usually triples
    c. length usually increases by 50%
    d. a and c above
    e. b and c above

4: Short-Answer Questions

1. Distinguish between five different states of arousal. Which state is optimal for breastfeeding? Why is this?

2. Briefly distinguish between Erikson's and Piaget's views of a toddler. Use at least two different elements to support your view.

3. Identify three different factors which have been related to childhood obesity. In what way is breastfeeding related to these factors?

4. Briefly discuss three developmental cues that infer readiness for solid foods.

5. Briefly discuss the phases of response which occur when a mother or father leaves a young child with strangers. Indicate ways in which a lactation consultant might interact with such a child without triggering "stranger anxiety."

6. How does a baby sleep? What implications does this have for the breastfeeding course?

7. Briefly distinguish between receptive and expressive language.

8. Define habituation. Give an example.

9. What is meant by cephalocaudal and proximaldistal growth?

5: Essay Questions

1.   Discuss four reflexes that are most likely to be present in the first few months of an infant's life. In each case indicate how they relate to breastfeeding behavior.

2.   Characterize an "easy" child, a "slow-to-warm-up" child, and a "difficult" child with regard to each of the following factors:
     a.   adapting to a change in routine
     b.   a positive or negative mood
     c.   attention span
     d.   distractability
     e.   sensory threshold
     For each factor, provide a breastfeeding-related example.

3.   Infant behaviors, including those related to breastfeeding, change over time. Select five different ages. For each age period indicate at least three typical behaviors of a child that age, including one related to breastfeeding.

4.   Explain why solid foods should be delayed until the second half of the first year of life.

5.   Attachment has been discussed as a process in which both parent and child participate. Discuss how a baby cues a parent to engage in appropriate nurturing behavior. Discuss how a parent cues a baby to be appropriately responsive.

6: Story Problem

You are asked to teach a growth and development class to high school sophomores.

1.   Indicate how you would illustrate how a baby grows.

2.   Relate such growth to feeding behavior.

A student asks you to distinguish between the importance of nature vs. nurture in producing a healthy child who grows to healthy adulthood.

3.   Do so.

One student protests: "But you never mentioned formula-feeding. Does that mean that my mother, who formula-fed me, didn't provide a healthy environment?"

4.   How do you answer her question?

Another student asks you if rooming-in is all that important, especially since women stay in hospitals for such a short time today: "Wouldn't it just be better if they got as much rest as possible and worry about the baby when they get home?"

5.   How do you respond to his concerns?

Another student approaches you after class and tells you that his baby sister died after being given an immunization. He questions whether such shots are all that necessary now that most childhood diseases don't exist anymore.

6.   Your response, please.

The last question from the class relates to dental health and breastfeeding.

7.   How do you respond to the teacher's request that you define nursing-bottle caries and how breastfed babies are at risk for this problem?

18

The Ill Breastfeeding Child

1: Outline of the Chapter

Infections
    Gastrointestinal
    Respiratory
    Meningitis
    Otitis media
Alteration in neurologic functioning
    Down syndrome
    Myelomeningocele
    Hydrocephalus
    Clinical implications
Congenital defects
    Congenital heart defects
    Oral and gastrointestinal defects
    Clinical implications
Metabolic dysfunction
    Inborn errors of metabolism
    Congenital hypothyroidism
    Celiac disease
    Cystic fibrosis
Allergies and food intolerance
    Allergies while breastfeeding
Hypoglycemia
Sudden infant death syndrome (SIDS)
Hospitalization
    Parental stresses
    Coping with siblings
    Emergency admission
    Home, the rebound effects

Chronic grief and loss
  The magic-milk syndrome
Empty cradle
Clinical implications
Summary

2: List of Key Concepts in the Chapter

The reader is urged to look for these key concepts in the body of the chapter and to develop questions deriving from these concepts as one way to gain understanding and insight into their relationship to lactation and breastfeeding. In this chapter, the reader is asked to compare the breastfeeding course of a healthy infant with that of one who is ill. Insight can be gained by distinguishing between an infant with an acute illness and an infant with a chronic condition. Attention should also be paid to how infant illness affects the maternal lactation course and overall parenting patterns.

Allergies
Celiac disease
Choanal atresia
Cleft lip/palate
Congenital heart defects
Congenital hypothyroidism
Cystic fibrosis
Down syndrome
Esophageal reflux
Galactosemia
Gastrointestinal infection
Grief
Hospitalization
Hydrocephalus
Hypoglycemia
Imperforate anus
Inborn errors of metabolism
"Magic milk" syndrome
Meningitis
Myelomeningocele
Otitis media
Pyloric stenosis
Respiratory infection
Sudden infant death syndrome (SIDS)
Tracheoesophageal fistula

3: Multiple-Choice Questions

1. Hospital admissions for which of the following illnesses are more likely for artificially fed infants when compared with breastfed infants?
   a. respiratory disease
   b. gastroenteritis
   c. other acute infections
   d. all of the above
   e. b and c above

2. Sudden infant death syndrome:
   a. is usually a diagnosis that is unconfirmed until autopsy
   b. never occurs in breastfeeding babies
   c. nearly always results in maternal engorgement
   d. a and c above
   e. none of the above

3. Food allergies in the breastfeeding infant:
   a. are nearly always traced to high-protein solid foods such as nuts or meat
   b. can be reduced if solid foods are not introduced for at least six months
   c. are often related to the maternal diet
   d. all of the above
   e. b and c above

4. Which of the following is a contraindication to breastfeeding by an affected infant?
   a. galactosemia
   b. cystic fibrosis
   c. PKU
   d. none of the above

5. Which of the following is an indication of dehydration?
   a. depressed anterior fontanel
   b. dry mucous membranes
   c. very warm extremities
   d. all of the above
   e. a and b above

4: Short-Answer Questions

1. Briefly identify at least five different foods that are associated with allergic reactions in infants and/or young children. Indicate in what foods they are most likely to be found.

2. Briefly discuss the rationale behind very early repair of a cleft lip. Include in your answer such factors as length of hospital stay, weight gain, and consideration of the repair site.

3. What is the "magic milk" syndrome? How might it impair a family's grief process? How might it help the parents to cope?

4. Briefly explain why oral glucose water should <u>not</u> be given to the hypoglycemic neonate.

5. Distinguish between a food allergy, food intolerance, and food sensitivity.

6. What is celiac disease and how is it related to infant feeding patterns?

7. What is congenital hypothyroidism? How might breastfeeding alter the course of the disease?

8. What is phenylketonuria and how is it related to breastfeeding?

9. Outline ways to prepare a young child for surgery. In what way(s) might such preparation be different for a baby/young child receiving human milk?

10. Briefly explain how the "dancer hand" position might assist a mother who is breastfeeding an ill infant or young child.

11. Upper respiratory illnesses can affect a baby's desire to feed. Briefly explain what is meant by this statement and what you might tell a mother whose baby has such an illness.

5: Essay Questions

1. Identify at least five principles of care during the hospitalization of a baby with a serious respiratory illness.

2. Explain how hospitalization can disrupt the life experience of a breastfeeding family. Indicate how such disruption can be minimized.

3. Your client's baby has been diagnosed with cystic fibrosis at 15 months of age–two months after weaning completely from the breast. What do you tell her when she asks if breastfeeding had anything to do with the baby's disease?

4. Identify each of the following problems and then discuss how it relates to oral feedings generally and to breastfeeding specifically:
   a. choanal atresia
   b. cleft palate
   c. tracheoesophageal fistula (T-E fistula)
   d. pyloric stenosis
   e. imperforate anus
   e. esophageal reflux

5. Explain how breastfeeding may be affected when a child is born with each of the following conditions:
   a. Down syndrome
   b. Hydrocephalus
   c. Myelomeningocele

6: Story Problem

The city where you live is experiencing an epidemic of upper respiratory illness, sometimes requiring hospitalization. Few of your breastfeeding clients have reported that their breastfeeding infants have been affected.

1. How do you explain this phenomenon to a class of pregnant couples who have expressed concern about giving birth in the midst of this epidemic?

One of your clients calls and asks if you feel she should bring her baby to the doctor. The child has refused to nurse and seems lethargic. In all other respects he seems normal to the mother.

2. What is your response to her?

Another one of your clients has just given birth to a baby with Down syndrome.

3. What do you tell her about the baby's ability to breastfeed when she asks if she can continue to feed her as she has her other five children?

A sick baby is seen by his doctor, who immediately admits him to the pediatric unit of the local hospital. The mother calls you, distraught that the nurses on the unit assume he is bottle-fed and are upset that he has refused to accept a bottle.

4. What do you advise the mother?

At the mother's insistence, a nurse from the hospital calls you. It is clear from her tone that she is contacting you under duress and would prefer not to be involved.

5. What do you tell her about this mother and her three-month-old infant who is exclusively breastfed?

The baby in question has been placed in a croupette to assist his breathing. When you see the mother, she is exhausted from worry and is unable to sleep on the fold-out chair that is in the baby's room. Her husband just called for news about the baby; during their conversation he mentions that their two older children, one of whom is a preschooler, are very upset at their mother's absence.

6. How do you help the mother to feel able to cope with her simultaneous desire to remain with her baby and her guilt at not being with her other children?

7. How do you help her to manage some of the difficulties of continued milk production in the face of her baby's distress and disinterest in breastfeeding; her increasingly full breasts; her difficulty expressing milk using a hand pump with a bulb syringe that the nurses have provided her; and her general exhaustion?

The mother's baby has been in the hospital for four days. On the first night the mother chooses not to stay at the hospital with her baby, he dies suddenly.

8. When her husband calls to tell you this, what four suggestions do you offer to help this family cope with their grief and loss? In your answer, be sure to discuss what you might share with the parents about how to help each other, as well as their remaining children.

19

Slow Weight Gain and Failure to Thrive

1: Outline of the Chapter

Normal growth
Growth charts
The slow-gaining infant
Failure to thrive (FTT)
Factors associated with inadequate caloric intake
    Management factors
    Infant factors
    Maternal factors
Clinical implications
    Devices for supplementation
    Other methods
Summary

2: List of Key Concepts in the Chapter

The reader is urged to look for these key concepts in the body of the chapter and to develop questions deriving from these concepts as one way to gain understanding and insight into their relationship to lactation and breastfeeding. Pay attention to the similarities and differences between a healthy, slow-gaining infant and one who is failing to thrive. Noting important cues in a careful history and observing a breastfeeding encounter help determine the diagnosis and how best to support an optimal breastfeeding course.

Disorganized suckling
Failure to thrive
Growth charts
Hypothyroidism

Inadequate caloric intake
Insufficient feedings
Insufficient glandular tissue
Neurologic dysfunction
Normal growth
Positioning
Slow-gaining
Supplementation devices
Tongue-tie

3: Multiple-Choice Questions

1. Which of the following drugs has been used to build up a low maternal milk supply?
    a. metoclopramide
    b. chlorindione
    c. ciprofloxacin
    d. chloramphenicol

2. According to the authors, a baby with a disorganized suckle:
    a. is usually one month of age or younger
    b. requires careful digital training to learn how to strip the lactiferous sinuses
    c. was often born prematurely
    d. all of the above
    e. a and c above

3. Insufficient glandular tissue is a problem:
    a. for approximately 50% of women in the developed world
    b. that explains nearly all infant failure to thrive
    c. that is relatively rare
    d. that is secondary to the use of antihistamines
    e. a and b above

4. Approximately what percentage of infants have been found to be gaining weight poorly as a result of an underlying organic problem?
    a. 85%
    b. 60%
    c. 40%
    d. 20%
    e. 5% or fewer

4: Short-Answer Questions

1. What is tongue-tie? How do you identify it?

2. Please explain the relationship of each of the following to inadequate infant weight gain and what you would recommend to clients:
   a. improper positioning
   b. insufficient numbers of feedings
   c. limited feeding length
   d. maternal hypothyroidism
   e. oral contraceptives and sedatives

3. Distinguish between infants with transitory and long-lasting neurologic difficulties and how   each might affect the breastfeeding course.

4. Briefly explain why detecting swallowing is important when attempting to determine the cause(s) of infant failure to thrive.

5. What is the relationship between infant weight gain and maternal milk production. Offer two examples–one of which suggests that the baby's suckling prompted inadequate milk production and one of which suggests that the mother's milk production was inadequate to sustain appropriate infant growth.

6. As a rule of thumb, what are two indicators of poor weight gain in a breastfeeding baby?

7. Briefly explain the role of genetic tendencies in patterns of infant weight gain. Please provide two different examples to support your answer.

8. Briefly define how one would conclude that a baby is gaining weight slowly, but is not failing to thrive.

5: Essay Questions

1. Identify at least four conditions that can result in infant failure to thrive. In each case identify how each might be identified and develop a plan of care for the breastfeeding mother.

2. What is a "flutter suck" and how does it relate to poor weight gain in the baby?

3. Explain how growth charts were devised and why they are sometimes considered problematic when evaluating growth patterns in breastfed infants.

4. Briefly describe what is considered a "normal" pattern of growth in a human infant, paying attention to three different indices of growth.

6: Story Problem

A client with a five-week-old infant is referred for evaluation of inadequate infant weight gain. The referring physician's note includes the following information:

Baby boy Jones was born following an uneventful pregnancy to a 28-year-old primipara who claims to be breastfeeding "on demand." Birth weight was 6 lbs., 14 oz.; weight at four weeks was 6 lbs., 2 oz. Length at birth was 19"; length at four weeks was 19-1/2". Maternal behavior is inconsistent with infant neglect. Evaluation for organic disease is negative.

1. Based on the above information, what do you suspect?

During your first appointment with the mother you take a history.

2. Based on that history, identify at least two different management issues which may have contributed to this baby's pattern of weight loss. Indicate how you have identified these issues and what intervention(s) you might recommend to overcome them.

3. Identify two additional maternal factors which may be implicated in this situation. Indicate how you have identified these factors and what intervention(s) you recommend to overcome them.

4. Identify two other infant factors which may be contributing to the baby's poor weight gain. Indicate how you have identified these factors and what intervention(s) you recommend to overcome them.

After taking the history, you ask the mother to breastfeed. Her baby has remained alert and quiet–with occasional fussing but was quieted by use of a pacifier during the 90 minutes of history-taking and discussion.

5. Describe <u>how</u> the mother brings her baby to the breast.

6. Describe <u>how</u> the infant suckles.

7. After observing the mother and baby breastfeeding, you suspect you know why the baby is gaining weight poorly. Explain what you observed that suggests an explanation.

8. Tell us what you then say to the mother to help her understand why her baby is gaining weight poorly.

9. Now indicate why you rule out a diagnosis of normal slow weight gain and conclude that the baby is failing to thrive.

You offer the mother several suggestions about how to get extra milk into the baby.

10. How does she respond to each of the following alternatives?
     a. a bottle after every breastfeeding
     b. cup-feeding after every breastfeeding
     c. spoon-feeding after every breastfeeding
     d. pumping her breasts
     e. breastfeeding the baby at least once (more) at night than has been occurring
     f. using a feeding tube device

11. About how much milk per feeding do you suggest that the mother put in the feeding tube device or other container she is using to give the baby extra fluid?

12. How do you answer the mother when she insists on knowing when she can "go back to just breastfeeding whenever Johnnie wants to"?

SECTION

FIVE

Contemporary Issues

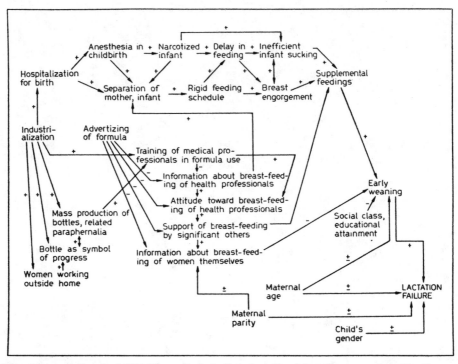

From Figure 1, Auerbach KG: The ecological, clinical, and sociological aspects of world-wide lactation failure, pp. 415-418; in Hirsch H, ed: The Family, Fourth International Congress of Psychosomatic Obstetrics and Gynecology, Tel Aviv, 1974 (Karger:Basel 1975).

20

Work Strategies and the Lactation Consultant

1: Outline of the Chapter

History
Certification
Developing a lactation program
    Playing politics
    The unique characteristics of breastfeeding counseling
    Assertiveness
Roles and responsibilities
    LCs and voluntary counselors
Marketing
Networking
Reporting and charting
    Nursing diagnosis
    Methods of charting
    Clinical care plans
Legal considerations
    Liability coverage
    Reimbursements
Private practice
    Why go into private practice?
    Setting up the practice
    The business of doing business
    Contact with other health-care workers
    Hospital privileges
    Problems in private practice
    The bottom line: why do they do It?
Do's and don'ts of lactation consulting
Summary

2: List of Key Concepts in the Chapter

The reader is urged to look for these key concepts in the body of the chapter and to develop questions deriving from these concepts as one way to gain understanding and insight into their relationship to lactation and breastfeeding. In this chapter, the attention of the reader is called to the similarities in development between lactation consultation as an allied health profession and the medical profession—which also developed out of a mentoring and apprenticeship form of training in advance of the availability of formalized academic training at a university. The reader may wish to compare the activities of lactation consultants with those of other health-care workers, noting both the commonalities and those areas where divergences occur.

Assertiveness
Burnout
Cash flow
Certification
Charting
Hospital privileges
Lactation consulting
Legal liability
Partnership
Politics
Rounds

3: Multiple-Choice Questions

1. When working with women co-workers, it is best to:
   a. be friendly
   b. attempt to become close friends
   c. accept and love yourself
   d. a and c above
   e. all of the above

2. Licensure is:
   a. governed by an agency of the federal government
   b. prohibits nonlicensed individuals from legally practicing the trade in question
   c. infers a minimum level of professional competence from licensed individuals
   d. b and c above
   e. all of the above

3. A health-care provider who is supportive of lactation services usually:
    a. has had a positive breastfeeding experience or is a father of breastfed children
    b. is a medical school graduate from the 1940s or 1950s
    c. has a well established practice and thus can "experiment" with something new
    d. b and c above
    e. all of the above

4. The history of lactation consulting reveals that it:
    a. developed when physicians recognized that its time intensive nature was more than they could provide
    b. developed when licensing boards recognized that certification was a more appropriate avenue to assess minimal competency
    c. developed out of the voluntary assistance provided by women to other women who sought to offer care within, as well as adjunct to, other health-care services
    d. a and b above
    e. all of the above

4: Short-Answer Questions

1. Briefly distinguish between a lactation consultant and a voluntary breastfeeding counselor.

2. Define assertiveness as it is used in this chapter. Briefly note how it differs from aggressiveness as a means of reaching a goal or solving a problem.

3. Identify the target audience for each of the following potential referral sources. Note which group is most likely to be the best advertisement and why:
    a. physicians
    b. mothers
    c. office nurses
    d. the general community

4. Distinguish between a solo practice and a partnership by noting five differences between the two.

5. What elements of a hospital-based lactation program can also be engaged in by an LC in private practice? Which elements should be limited to a hospital-based program?

6. Define burnout. Offer an example of how it can occur.

7.   Identify three problems relating to private lactation consulting. Indicate how each might be resolved or prevented from occurring in the first place.

8.   Briefly discuss each of the following legal issues. Include in your discussion an example that clearly avoids the legal problem in question.
   a.   permission to touch
   b.   avoiding a guarantee
   c.   avoiding causing emotional distress
   d.   confidentiality of information

5: Essay Questions

1.   What is problem-oriented medical record-keeping? Provide a brief example focusing on some aspect of breastfeeding. Indicate at least two different ways which this method of charting can serve:
   a.   when the LC works in a physician's office
   b.   when the LC works in a hospital
   c.   when the LC maintains a private practice

2.   Identify four advantages and four disadvantages to incorporation for a practice in lactation consulting. In each case, note how an advantage might become a disadvantage and how a disadvantage might be changed into an advantage.

3.   Read Table 20-1: "IBLCE Examination Summary Data, 1985-1991." Based on the information provided, offer a brief overview characterizing the certification outcomes for the entire group of certification candidates.

4.   Identify which health-care providers should work together to assist the lactating mother of a breastfeeding baby who has failed to regain birth weight at one month of age. Explain how each person can provide assistance and in what way(s) they need to communicate with one another to effect optimal care in both the short- and long-term.

6: Story Problem

You are a lactation consultant new to the town.

1.   Indicate your credentials, if any, where your practice is located, and how you introduced yourself to both the health-care community and the community at large.

You see the president of the local medical society one evening. He turns away from you with a scowl on his face.

2.   What do you do? Why?

Later that week, you receive a letter indicating that your application for hospital privileges has been turned down.

3.   What do you do? Why?

You have been working as a lactation consultant for three months. The two medical practices whose clients you serve as a prenatal breastfeeding educator have expanded. You are having difficulty meeting the needs of their pregnant clients and seeing them postpartum.

4.   What three alternatives do you suggest to the physicians in these two practices? Why?

You have been in practice for 15 months. One morning you walk into a physician's office to see a client, and the clinic manager whispers to you that a move is afoot to deny you access to clients. Apparently another physician has complained to the medical staff that you are "practicing medicine without a license."

5.   How do you handle this?

Three more years have passed. At last night's medical staff meeting of the largest pediatric clinic in town–a practice you have served since your arrival–you receive a standing ovation for your tireless work with their clients. The founding member of the clinic hands you a bouquet of red roses, kisses you on the cheek, and pats your derriere.

6.   What do you do when they ask you to "say a few words"?

21

Research and Breastfeeding

1: Outline of the Chapter

2: List of Key Concepts in the Chapter

The reader is urged to look for these key concepts in the body of the chapter and to develop questions deriving from these concepts as one way to gain understanding and insight into their relationship to lactation and breastfeeding. In this chapter, attention should be paid to the issues relating to the use of breastfeeding babies, lactating mothers, and human milk samples in a wide variety of research endeavors. When considering a research question, ask yourself whether sufficient attention has been paid to avoiding intrusion into the breastfeeding relationship–so that maternal milk production and/or infant behavior at the breast is not compromised. The reader may find that a careful review of these chapter elements highlights the many research questions that need to be asked–and which can be answered without harming the relationship the reader is seeking to understand more clearly.

Data analysis
Data collection
Ethnography
Grounded theory
Hypotheses
Methodology
Operational definitions
Phenomenology
Population
Quantitative and qualitative approaches
Reliability
Research problem, purpose
Review of literature
Rights of human subjects
Sampling
Setting
Validity
Variables

3: Multiple-Choice Questions

1. Grounded theory refers to:
    a. a method used to understand beliefs, practices, and behavior patterns within the context of a particular culture or subculture
    b. a method that focuses attention on those behaviors occurring on dirt floors

    c. a method that generates a theory explaining an action within a particular social context

    d. a method designed to understand the meaning of life experiences from the perspective of those who are living the experience under study

2. An experimental study requires careful control of:
    a. the treatment
    b. the subject groups
    c. randomization of subjects within the study groups
    d. b and c above
    e. all of the above

3. The variable that changes the action of a dependent variable is:
    a. a confounding variable
    b. an intervening variable
    c. an independent variable
    d. all of the above
    e. a and b above

4. When a researcher chooses to write a null hypothesis, this means that:
    a. the relationship between the dependent and independent variables is found to be null and void upon testing
    b. the statement is written to predict no difference in the dependent variable by the action of the independent variable
    c. the statement is written to predict a significant difference in the dependent variable only if at least two intervening variables also change
    d. the relationship between the dependent and the independent variables is secondary to the relationship between the independent variable and at least two confounding variables

4: Short-Answer Questions

1. Briefly define and distinguish between qualitative and quantitative research methods. Provide one example of a research question appropriate to each approach.

2. Briefly distinguish between descriptive, correlational, and experimental studies. Give an example of a research question appropriate to each type of study.

3. What is a quasi-experimental study?

4. How might triangulation be used to strengthen the findings of a research study?

5. What is the importance of the rights of human subjects in a research study? How are these rights protected if the subject in question is:
    a. the lactating mother?
    b. the breastfeeding baby?
    c. milk samples from several lactating mothers?

6. Briefly distinguish between a dependent and an independent variable.

7. What is an operational definition? Give an example.

8. Briefly distinguish between the purpose of a review of literature for a qualitative study and a review of literature for a quantitative study.

9. What is the difference between probability and nonprobability sampling? Give an example of each.

10. What is the difference between reliability and validity? Why is each important?

5: Essay Questions

1. What elements are part of a quantitative method? In what sense are such methods considered to be "objective"?

2. What are the four basic rights of human subjects as determined by the Nuremberg Code? How might each relate to a study involving lactating mothers and/or their breastfeeding infants?

3. Distinguish among simple random sampling, systematic sampling, stratified random sampling, a sample of convenience, snowball sampling, and solicited sampling. Which is considered the most rigorous? Why?

4. Indicate when each of the following data collection techniques might be used. Give an   example of a research question relating to breastfeeding which would be amenable to each technique:
    a. self-report questionnaire
    b. interview (face-to-face or telephone)
    c. observation (both when the subject is aware of the observation and when the subject is not)
    d. biophysiologic measurement

5. In what way(s) might you determine that a research report is relevant to your work as a clinician?

6. How might researchers and clinicians work together to increase the likelihood that the research questions being posed are relevant to clinicians and the answers deriving from research endeavors can be used by clinicians?

6: Story Problem

You have been asked to design a study relating to lactation.

1. What research question have you decided to ask?

2. What is the research problem underlying the research question?

3. Who/what will serve as your research subject(s)?

4. What is the purpose of the study?

5. In what way(s) do you think this study will help other research investigators— as well as lactation consultants and other health-care workers in clinical practice?

6. Outline the elements you would include in a consent form for this study.

7. What kind of sampling would you need to do?

8. What is your sample population?

9. How would you obtain your sample population?

10. If you plan to compare two or more groups, how do you distinguish between each group so that they are truly "discrete"?

11. How will you determine the reliability of the data you collect? Its validity? Its internal consistency?

12. What kind(s) of statistics will you use to analyze the data you have collected?

13. What is your most important finding? What two other findings will you discuss?

14. Indicate how the findings identified in question 13 above could be used by clinicians working with breastfeeding mothers and babies in both an outpatient and a hospital setting. In what way(s) might these findings also generate additional research?

22

Issues in Human Milk Banking

1: Outline of the Chapter

History of human milk banking
Cultural issues
Clinical uses
Current practice
    Donor selection and screening
    Heat treatment
    Packaging for heat treatment
    Collection, handling, and storage
    Packaging and transport
    Future technological challenges
Quality assurance
    Bacterial screening
    Environmental pollutants
    Policies and procedures
Cost containment and survival
Marketing strategies
Summary

2: List of Key Concepts in the Chapter

The reader is urged to look for these key concepts in the body of the chapter and to develop questions deriving from these concepts as one way to gain understanding and insight into their relationship to lactation and breastfeeding. In this chapter, attention should be paid not only to the history of human milk banking and its implications for product use today, but also to current concerns relating to donor selection, screening, handling of the milk, and quality assurance–and how human milk banking is likely to change in an era of heightened fear of bacterial and viral pandemics.

Banked human milk
Cultural issues
Donors of human milk
Environmental pollutants
Heat treatment
Marketing banked human milk
Milk collection
Milk handling
Milk screening
Milk storage
Quality assurance procedures

3: Multiple-Choice Questions

1. Human milk banks are a product of the:
    a. late twentieth century
    b. late nineteenth century
    c. early twentieth century
    d. late eighteenth century

2. Milk bank donors are:
    a. sometimes paid
    b. healthy
    c. not using drugs or over-the-counter medications
    d. b and c above
    e. all of the above

3. Bacteriological screening of raw human milk has revealed that:
    a. premature infants are at significantly increased risk of sepsis when bacterio-
        logical counts in such milk are high
    b. infants fed raw milk often receive high levels of coagulase-negative staphy-
        lococci
    c. the risk of sepsis from the ingestion of raw human milk is very low
    d. all of the above
    e. b and c above

4. Pasteurization of human milk is most likely to affect:
    a. vitamins
    b. lipids
    c. niacin
    d. riboflavin
    e. EGF

4: Short-Answer Questions

1. Briefly explain why describing breastmilk as a form of altered blood may not be viewed as appropriate.

2. What is a graft vs. host reaction? How does it relate to donor milk?

3. Briefly explain why most banked milk is stored in pooled batches.

4. What do the FDA and CDC recommend regarding the heat treatment of banked human milk? Why is this important?

5. Briefly explain what lacto-engineering is and how it might affect banked human milk.

6. What is quality assurance and how is it incorporated into human milk bank procedures?

7. Briefly explain why environmental contamination is an issue for human milk banks.

8. What is a "kitchen" milk bank and how may it be at-risk for continued operation?

5: Essay Questions

1. Explain when donor milk might be used in a neonatal intensive care unit. Why is this not a universal practice in all NICUs?

2. What is the relationship between necrotizing enterocolitis, IgA deficiency, malabsorption syndrome, severe burns, inborn errors of metabolism, and banked human milk feedings?

3. How do each of the following affect banked human milk?
   a. heat treatment
   b. freezing
   c. handling
   d. packaging

4. Identify at least eight conditions for excluding potential breastmilk donors from offering their milk to a milk bank. Indicate whether each would be temporary or permanent.

6: Story Problem

You have been asked to provide instructions to a mother who wishes to donate her milk to a milk bank at her local hospital.

1. What do you tell this mother after she informs you that the hospital milk bank representative is out sick and that the donor mother has been asked to provide milk tomorrow?

2. Explain to the mother at least seven different situations in which her milk may be used.

The mother calls you and is indignant that she has been asked questions about HIV risk factors.

3. What do you tell her?

A local newspaper calls to ask for an interview about human milk banking in the era of AIDS.

4. How do you reply to the reporter's insistence in viewing human milk as a "carrier" of HIV?

A client from your practice is unable to totally nourish her baby on breastmilk following an auto accident in which she sustained injuries requiring extensive surgery on her upper chest. Her baby has responded poorly to all artificial baby milks offered. Your client asks if banked human milk, which the baby's pediatric gastroenterologist has suggested trying, is safe to use.

5. What is your reply?

6. What do you explain to her about how the milk is treated and what its effects might be on her baby?

The baby is now thriving; however, her intake is such that the milk bank coordinator is concerned about how long the local bank can continue to supply milk.

7. What do you suggest to the mother?

Answers To Multiple-choice Questions

Chapter 1	Chapter 6	Chapter 11	Chapter 16	Chapter 21
1. c	1. a	1. a	1. b	1. c
2. d	2. c	2. b	2. c	2. e
3. a	3. d	3. d	3. b	3. d
4. d	4. c	4. c	4. e	4. b

Chapter 2	Chapter 7	Chapter 12	Chapter 17	Chapter 22
1. c	1. e	1. d	1. e	1. c
2. e	2. a	2. e	2. a	2. e
3. d	3. c	3. b	3. d	3. e
4. b	4. d	4. e	4. b	4. b
5. a			5. e	

Chapter 3	Chapter 8	Chapter 13	Chapter 18
1. c	1. a	1. b	1. d
2. a	2. d	2. c	2. d
3. b	3. c	3. a	3. c
4. a	4. b	4. c	4. a
		5. e	5. e

Chapter 4	Chapter 9	Chapter 14	Chapter 19
1. b	1. a	1. c	1. a
2. c	2. e	2. a	2. e
3. a	3. b	3. c	3. c
4. c	4. e	4. a	4. d
	5. d		

Chapter 5	Chapter 10	Chapter 15	Chapter 20
1. a	1. d	1. e	1. d
2. b	2. b	2. b	2. d
3. b	3. c	3. b	3. a
	4. d	4. d	4. c

STUDY QUESTIONS PERTAINING TO THE APPENDICES TO

Breastfeeding and Human Lactation

Appendix A: <u>Sample Breastfeeding Policies and Protocols</u>

1. Your hospital has adopted the St. Joseph Medical Center Breastfeeding Policies. However, the original chairman of the Breastfeeding Policies and Protocols Committee, an individual who was instrumental in getting the policies adopted, has been replaced. The new chairman is an individual who never was supportive of such a change. Provide a justification for each of the 17 policies to convince the new chairman that the Policies should stand.

2. Select one technique by which health-care providers at your institution will make a functional assessment of the infant at the breast.
    a. Identify <u>why</u> you have selected this particular technique.
    b. Explain <u>how</u> you will teach this technique to staff nurses and house physicians who work with mothers and babies.
    c. Indicate <u>how</u> you will determine if this functional assessment:
        (1) identifies babies and mothers in need of additional assistance
        (2) identifies babies who are "nipple-confused."
    d. Explain <u>how</u> you will go about sharing what you have learned regarding this assessment technique with colleagues in your profession and other health-care workers   who assist breastfeeding mothers and babies.

3. Justify to a nurse manager why breastfeeding assessments require an average of 20 minutes–in a setting where nurse staffing has been severely eroded at the same time that your community has experienced a "birthing boomlet."

4. Explain how you would use a lactation consultant in a hospital where every nurse working with new mothers and babies has successfully completed a week-long training course designed to make them effective "lactation initiators."*

---

*Humenick, SS: A call for the lactation initiator: setting the standards (editorial), *J Hum Lact* 8:121, 1992.

5. Compare the breastfeeding policies from St. Joseph Medical Center and the Wellstart Lactation Program in San Diego. Identify similar individual policies from each set and compare them.
   a. How does each differ from the other? For example: How many times should a baby be offered the breast according to the St. Joseph policy? How does this relate to the recommendation pertaining to feeding frequency found in the Wellstart policy?
   b. Which differences suggest a need to rewrite that particular policy? If so, how would you recommend that it be rewritten, and why do you make this recommendation?
   c. Both policies provide supportive documentation for each of the policy statements. How would you support the selection of references? What criticisms might be offered?

6. Examine the St. Joseph Medical Center Family Birthplace Breastfeeding Education Protocol.
   a. An international evaluator of your maternity services is touring your unit and notes that you have developed the same breastfeeding education protocol that St. Joseph Medical Center uses. This visitor has several questions. Please provide a rebuttal to each of the following objections raised to the use of this protocol.
      (1) "Research has shown that undecided mothers are unimpressed with the benefits of human milk for babies as a reason for breastfeeding. Why do you bother with such information?"
      (2) "Your government gives away formula to poor mothers; therefore, the cost savings of breastfeeding is rendered moot. Why do you bother mentioning this as a benefit?"
      (3) "How can you say breastfeeding is 'convenient' when such a high proportion of new mothers in your city go back to work within a few weeks of their baby's birth? Surely, for them, bottle-feeding would be easier–if only because someone else can take responsibility for feeding the baby."
      (4) "If the mother can always change her mind and discontinue breastfeeding, aren't you admitting that modern formulas and breastmilk are equivalent and equally nutrititious for the human infant?"
      (5) "You are very short-staffed. Why is it necessary for the nurse to take valuable time with each patient when you have all of these patient education materials she can take home?"
      (6) "At our hospital, 'Kangaroo care' is practiced routinely in the NICU for as many babies as possible, including many who are less than 36 weeks gestation. We have found that these infants go to breast quite readily, often well in advance of 36 weeks. Given your insistence that

breastfeeding is so much better for term babies, aren't you contradicting yourself by not offering pre-terms the same opportunity to breastfeed–simply on the basis of their gestational age?"

(7)   "You seem to have many 'rules' for optimal breastfeeding. Why don't you simply stand back, with your hands in your pockets, and watch how mothers and babies do it without help?"

(8)   "Technology seems to be highly valued in the United States. What would you do if you didn't have those extremely expensive, fancy breast pumps?"

(9)   "Please tell me how you know that a lactating breast is 'empty'. I am unfamiliar with this concept."

(10)   "You do not seem to like mothers to supplement; however, many women do so and your food stores and other places seem to stock all manner of artificial feeding gadgets. Don't you think you are fighting a losing battle?"

(11)   "You place great importance on mothers getting rest, but babies need to eat, often on a schedule unrelated to others' needs. How can you provide for the mother's need to rest and at the same time see to it that the baby gets to breast when s/he is most receptive to suckling?"

(12)   "I have noticed that on other floors in the hospital–including pediatrics–gifts do not go home with the patients. However, on the maternity floor, much is made of the opportunity for the hospital to give the mothers and babies something, as if such a
gift will make them recall their experience more positively. Why do you think new mothers need such gifts?"

(13)   "Your answer to my previous question was very interesting. In my country, these 'gift packs' are simply not allowed in the hospital. Why don't you do that here?"

Appendix B: <u>Breastfeeding Assessment Record</u> <u>(St. Joseph Medical Center)</u>

Carefully examine the St. Joseph Medical Center Breasfeeding Assessment Record.

1.   How might you improve it?

2.   Provide a rationale for each of your recommendations for improvement.

Appendix C: <u>Nursing Diagnoses Related to Breastfeeding</u>

1. Examine the definitions for "Effective Breastfeeding," "Ineffective Breastfeeding," and "Interrupted Breastfeeding."
    a. How would you incorporate these definitions and their respective defining characteristics into documenting/charting breastfeeding in a hospital or clinic setting?
    b. In what way(s) might you improve on each of these definitions?
    c. In what way(s) might these definitions be influenced by the cultural/ethnic group to which the mothers you assist belong?

Appendix D: <u>New York State Code in Support of Breastfeeding</u>

1. How would you go about getting this Code adopted in your state/province?
    a. Whom would you approach first, next? Why would you choose these individuals?
    b. In what way(s) might the breastfeeding mothers in your state/province get involved in such an action plan?
    c. How might your professional association(s) get involved?
        (1) Which group(s) are these?
        (2) What kind of role might each take?
    d. How might knowledge of breastfeeding initiation and duration rates be helpful in your campaign to get a Code in Support of Breastfeeding adopted in your state/province?
    e. What about differences in breastfeeding initiation and duration by maternal ethnic/racial group, socioeconomic status, and other social factors?
    f. How might such a Code benefit the hospitals/maternity centers in your state/province?

2. Are any hospitals in your state/province identified as "baby friendly"? How might such a Code assist a hospital in your community in reaching a goal of baby friendliness?

3. How might such a state/province-wide Code assist in improving the care for breastfeeding mothers that currently characterizes the teaching centers in your state/province?

Appendix E: <u>Prototype Lactation Consultant Job Proposal or Description</u>

1. Describe YOUR job as a lactation consultant in a hospital/clinic. If you have a private practice, describe the services you offer clients.

2. In what way(s) does your job description support the need for such a service in your community?

3. If you work in a hospital, how does what you do before the mother is discharged assist her past the first week of her newborn's life?

4. In what way(s) does your job description include coordinating your services with those of other health-care professionals–in the hospital, in the community?
    a. If it does not, how might you alter your practice to provide such a link between the services you offer and those which are available from others?

5. In what way(s) do you participate in scholarly activities–e.g., reading the professional literature, engaging in research studies, and/or writing grant proposals?
    a. How might you increase the frequency with which you engage in one or more of theseactivities?
    b. How would this activity help you in your practice?

6. In what way(s) do you participate in programs–for the public or for other professionals–about lactation and breastfeeding?
    a. How might you increase the frequency with which you engage in these activities?
    b. How would this activity help you in your practice?

Appendix F: <u>Recommendations and Competencies for Lactation Consultant Practice</u>

1. How might you use such a document to encourage the development of a lactation consultant service in a local medical center/clinic?

or

2. How might you use such a document to highlight the services you provide as a lactation consultant?

3. In what way(s) could you increase your own competency through a review of the competencies listed in the text of Appendix F?

Appendix G: <u>Breastfeeding Support Resources</u>

1. How could you use this listing?

2. What does this listing tell you?
    a. About professional associations pertaining to breastfeeding?
    b. About mother-to-mother support groups worldwide?

3. Identify three breastfeeding support groups from your own country.
    a. How would you describe each of these groups? Are they for professionals or for mothers?
    b. What might you gain from contact with each of these groups?

4. Select a country other than your own. How would you characterize the groups represented in this country?

Appendix H: <u>Tables of Equivalents and Methods of Conversion</u>

1. Explain how you would use this Table of Equivalents in your daily practice.
    a. Why are such equivalents and conversion methods important to clinical practice?

2. Do you have a method of checking equivalents when working with a mother?
    a. What method/technique do you use? Why?

Appendix I: <u>Wellstart Patient History</u>

1. Evaluate this patient history form.
    a. What are its strengths?
    b. In what way(s) do you feel it might be improved?
    c. How conveniently is it structured for clinical use?
    d. What elements might you add? Why?

2. What portion(s) of this patient history would you be <u>least</u> likely to use? Why?

3. What portion(s) of this patient history would you be <u>most</u> likely to use? Why?

Appendix J: <u>Conversion Tables</u>

1. Do you use such tables in your practice now? Why or why not?

2. When might such conversion tables come in handy?

Appendix K: <u>Critical Care Plan</u>

1. Examine this care plan for the breastfeeding couple following a vaginal birth.

2. How might you apply it when:
    a. the mother has had her first baby, her family is adamantly opposed to her breastfeeding, but she has a history of severe allergies and wants to protect her baby from similar difficulties?
    b. the mother has just given birth to her sixth child. At home, she has an 18-month-old, four-year-old twins, a six-year-old, and a nine-year-old. She breastfed her first two children, but not her most recent three. She is thinking about breastfeeding this "last" baby.
    c. the mother has just given birth to her second baby (her first child is now three years old), and she is planning to return to work full-time within four weeks. Her husband recently lost his job, they moved into a new home six months ago, and both are worried about making the payments on only one income. She breastfed her first baby for two months and quit when she returned to work. She has just confided to you that she "hates" the idea of using a breast pump.

3. For each of the cases outlined above:
    a. Develop a daily care plan designed to optimize each mother's in-hospital breastfeeding experience.
    b. Develop a discharge plan that takes into consideration the information provided above.
    c. Identify what breastfeeding pamphlets you will recommend and how they will support your one-on-one teaching plan.
    d. Will you invite this mother to view a video about breastfeeding? If so, which one? Why that particular item?
    e. What kind of community support can you offer this mother?

4. Finally, what is your assessment of each mother's likely breastfeeding course? How might it be extended? What factors might shorten her breastfeeding course?

GLOSSARY OF TERMS FOUND IN
Breastfeeding and Human Lactation

Acinus Smallest division of a gland; a group of secretory cells arrayed around a central cavity. In the breast, an acinus secretes milk. Acini (pl). *See also*: alveolus.

Aerobic Requiring air for metabolic processes, e.g., aerobic bacteria. Normal skin, including the breast, is colonized with aerobic bacteria.

Afferent Being conducted toward an organ or gland. Suckling produces afferent impulses which travel from the nipple to the pituitary gland, which then releases oxytocin causing milk to let down. The opposite of efferent.

Allergen Any substance causing an allergic response. Foods, drugs, or inhalants may be allergens. Cow's milk protein is a common allergen of infants.

Alphalactalbumin The principal protein found in the whey portion of human milk; it assists the synthesis of lactose. The dominant whey protein in cow's milk and most artificial infant milks, betalactoglobulin, is not found in human milk. *See also*: Non-casein protein.

Alveolar ridge The ridge on the hard palate immediately behind the upper gums. Movement of the infant's jaw during nursing compresses the areola between his tongue and alveolar ridge.

Alveolus In the mammary gland, a small sac at the terminus of a lobule in which milk is secreted and stored. Alveoli (pl). Groups of alveoli, organized in lobes, give the mammary gland the appearance of a "bunch of grapes." *See also*: Acinus.

Ampulla A normally dilated portion of a duct. Ampullae (pl). Ampullae in the lactiferous ducts underlie the areola near the base of the nipple. *See also*: Lactiferous sinus.

Anorectal anomalies and abnormalities Anomalies of the rectum, the lower few inches of the large intestine, and the anus, the opening in the skin at the distal end of the rectum. An example is imperforate anus, in which the rectum ends in a blind pouch.

Antibody An immunoglobulin formed in response to an antigen, including bacteria and viruses. Antibodies then recognize and attack those bacteria or viruses, thus helping the body resist infection. Breastmilk contains antibodies to antigens to which either the mother or the infant have been exposed.

Antigen   A substance which stimulates antibody production. It may be introduced into the body (as dust, food, or bacteria) or produced within it (as a by-product toxin).

Antigenemia   The state of having an antigen of interest in the blood.

Areola   Pigmented skin surrounding the nipple which overlies the ampullae or lactiferous sinuses. In order to suckle effectively, an infant should have his gums placed well back on the areola.

Artificial infant milk   Any milk preparation, other than human milk, intended to be the sole nourishment of human infants.

Atopic eczema   An inherited allergic tendency to rashes or inflammation of the skin. Exclusively breastfed infants are less likely to manifest this condition, as cow's milk protein is a common allergen.

Atresia, intestinal   Congenital blockage or closure of any part of the intestinal tract.

Axilla   The underarm area; in it lies the uppermost extent of the mammary ridge or milk line. Deep breast tissue (the axillary tail or "tail of Spence") extends towards and sometimes into the axilla. This tissue may engorge the axilla along with the rest of the breast in the early postpartum.

B-cell   A lymphocyte produced in bone marrow and peripheral lymphoid tissue which is found in breastmilk. It attacks antigens and is one type of cell which confers cell-mediated immunity.

Bactericidal   Capable of destroying bacteria. Breastmilk contains so many bactericidal cells that the bacteria count of expressed milk actually declines during the first 36 hours following expression.

Bacteriostatic   Capable of inhibiting the proliferation of bacterial colonies.

BALT/GALT/MALT   Bronchus/Gut/Mammary-Associated Immunocompetent Lymphoid Tissue. A lymphocyte pathway which causes IgA antibodies to be produced in the mammary gland after a lactating woman is exposed to an antigen on her intestinal or respiratory mucosa. These antibodies are then transferred through breastmilk to the breastfeeding infant, who thus may possess antibodies to antigens to which he has not been directly exposed.

Banked human milk   *See: Don*or milk.

Betalactoglobulin   The dominant protein present in the whey fraction of the milk of cows and other ruminants; it is absent from human milk.

Bioavailable   That portion of an ingested nutrient actually absorbed and used by the body. Because the nutrients in breastmilk are highly bioavailable, low concentrations may actually result in more nutrients absorbed by the infant than do the higher, less bioavailable, concentrations in cow's milk or artificial infant milks.

Buccal pads   Fat pads sheathed by the masseter muscles in young infants' cheeks. The buccal pads touch and provide stability for the tongue, which enhances its ability to compress breast tissue during suckling. Breastfed infants typically have a plump-cheeked appearance because of well- developed buccal pads.

Candidiasis   A fungal infection caused by *Candida albicans* or "thrush." Common in the maternal vagina, it may inoculate the infant during delivery and be transferred from the infant's mouth to the mother's nipple. Candidiasis of the nipple and breast may produce intense nipple and breast pain. In the infant it may produce white spots on the oral mucosa and a bright red, painful rash ringing the anus. Formerly termed moniliasis.

Casein   The principal protein in milks of all mammals. Human milk has a ratio of soluble whey proteins to casein of about 65:35. Casein of human milk forms soft, easily digested curds in the infant stomach. The whey-to-casein ratio in cow's milk is 20:80; artificial infant milks have whey-to-casein ratios which vary from those of cow's milk to 40:60. Cow's milk casein forms firm curds which require a high expenditure of energy to digest.

Centers for Disease Control (CDC)   An agency of the United States Public Health Service established in 1973 to protect the public health of the nation by providing leadership and direction in the prevention and control of diseases and other preventable health conditions–and to respond to public health emergencies.

Certification   The process by which a nongovernmental professional association attests that an individual has met certain standards specified by the association for the practice of that profession.

Colostrum   The fluid in the breast at the end of pregnancy and in the early postpartum. It is thicker and yellower than mature milk, reflecting a higher content of proteins, many of which are immunoglobulins. It is also higher in fat-soluble vitamins (including A, E, and K) and some minerals (including sodium and zinc).

Congenital infection   An infection existing at birth which was acquired transplacentally. Infections which may be so acquired include HIV and TORCH organisms. *See also: H*uman Immunodeficiency Virus; TORCH.

Conjunctivitis   Inflammation of the mucous membrane that lines the eyelid. In many traditional and some modern societies, fresh breastmilk is instilled into the eyes to alleviate this condition.

Contraception   Preventing conception. Breastfeeding provides significant contraceptive protection during the first few months postpartum–as long as the infant is fully breastfed, feeds during the night, and maternal menses have not resumed.

Cooper's ligaments   Triangular, vertical ligaments in the breast which attach deeper layers of subcutaneous tissue to the skin.

Cord blood   Blood remaining in the umbilical cord after birth.

Creamatocrit   The proportion of cream in a milk sample determined by measuring the depth of the cream layer in a centrifuged sample. An indicator of caloric content of milk which must be used with care, the fat (and thus caloric) content of human milk varies between breasts, within a feed, diurnally, and over the entire course of lactation.

Cross nursing   Occasional wet-nursing on an informal, short-term basis, usually in the context of childcare.

Cytoprotective   Any condition or factor which protects cells from inflammation or death.

Diagnostic-related grouping (DRG)   A group of diagnoses for health conditions which result in similar intensity of hospital care and similar length of hosptial stay for patients hospitalized with those conditions.

Disaccharide   A carbohydrate composed of two monosaccharides. The principal sugar in human milk is lactose, a disaccharide; its constituent monosaccharides are glucose and galactose.

Donor milk   Human milk voluntarily contributed to a human milk bank by women unrelated to the recipient.

Donor milk, fresh-frozen   Fresh-raw milk that has been stored frozen at -20°C for less than 12 months.

Donor milk, fresh-raw   Milk stored continuously at 4°C for not longer than 72 hours after collection.

Donor milk, heat-treated   Fresh-raw milk or fresh-frozen milk which has been heated to a minimum of 56°C for 30 minutes.

Donor milk, pooled   A batch of milk which contains milk from more than one donor.

Dopamine   The "prolactin inhibiting factor" (PIF), or a mediator of the prolactin inhibiting factor, secreted in the hypothalamus. It blocks the release of prolactin into the bloodstream.

Drip milk   Milk that leaks from a breast which is not being directly stimulated. Since its fat content is low it should not be used regularly for infant feedings.

Ductules   Small ducts in the mammary gland which drain milk from the alveoli into larger lactiferous ducts that terminate in the nipple.

Dyad   A pair–e.g., the breastfeeding mother and her infant.

Eczema   Skin inflammation or rash. See also: Atopic eczema.

Elemental formula   Artificial infant milks containing fats, proteins, and carbohydrates in their simplest (most elemental) forms.

Eminences of the pars villosa   Tiny swellings on the inner surfaces of infant's lips which help theinfant to retain a grasp on the breast during suckling.

Energy density   The number of calories per unit volume; caloric density. Mature human milk averages 65 calories/100 ml, controlled largely by the fat content of the milk.

Envelope virus   A virus which requires its coat (envelope) to infect other cells. If the envelope is destroyed–e.g., by heat or soap and water–the ability of the virus to produce infection is destroyed. Cytomegalovirus and Human Immunodeficiency Virus are two envelope viruses.

Epidemiology   The study of the frequency and distribution of disease and the factors which cause that frequency and distribution.

Epiglottis   Cartilaginous structure of the larynx. An infant's epiglottis lies just below the soft palate. It closes the larynx when the infant swallows, ensuring passage of milk to the esophagus.

Estrogen   A hormone which causes growth of mammary tissue during part of each menstrual cycle, assists in the secretion of prolactin during pregnancy, and is one of the hormones whose concentration falls sharply at parturition.

Exogenous   Derived from outside the body–e.g., iron supplements which provide the infant with exogenous iron.

Foremilk   The milk obtained at the beginning of a breastfeed. Its higher water content keeps the infant hydrated and supplies water-soluble vitamins and proteins. Its fat content (1-2 gm/100 ml) is lower than that of hindmilk.

Frenulum   Fold of mucous membrane, midline on the underside of the tongue, which helps to anchor the tongue to the floor of the mouth. A short or inelastic frenulum, or one attached close to the tip of the tongue, may restrict tongue extension enough to inhibit effective breastfeeding. The frenum.

Fructose   A carbohydrate present in human milk in small quantities.

Galactorrhea   Abnormal production of milk. It may occur under psychological influences or be a sign of pituitary tumor.

Galactose   A monosaccharide present in small quantities in human milk. It is derived from lactose and in turn helps produce elements essential for the development of the human central nervous system.

Gastroenteritis   Inflammation of the stomach and intestines resulting from bacterial or viral invasion. Breastfed infants are at less risk of this illness.

Gastroschisis   An opening in the wall of the abdomen; a congenital malformation.

Gestational age   An infant's age since conception, usually specified in weeks. Counted from the first day of the last normal menstrual period.

Hindmilk   Milk released near the end of a breastfeed, after active let-down of milk. Fat content of hindmilk may rise to 6% or more, two or three times the concentration in foremilk.

Horizontal transmission   Transmission of pathogens through direct contact. *See also*: Vertical transmission.

Human Immunodeficiency Virus (HIV)   A retrovirus which disarms the body's immune system causing death from an opportunistic infection. First identified in 1981. The virus may be transmitted to unborn infants, and it is carried in the breastmilk, although not all breastfed infants born to HIV-positive mothers become ill themselves. The greatest risk to the infant is posed when a woman has her initial HIV-related illness while pregnant or breastfeeding.

Human milk   Milk secreted in the human breast.

Human milk bank   A service which collects, screens, processes, stores, and distributes donated human milk to meet the needs of those, usually infants, for whom human milk has been prescribed by a physician.

Human milk fortifiers   Nutrients added to expressed human milk in order to enhance the growth and nutrient balances of very low-birth-weight infants. Added protein may be derived from protein components of donor human milk or from cow's-milk-based products. See also: Lactoengineering.

Hydration   The water balance within a body. Adequate hydration is necessary to maintain normal body temperature and for most other metabolic functions. Breastmilk is 90% water. Therefore, even in hot or dry climates, a fully breastfed infant obtains all the water he requires through breastmilk.

Hyperalimentation   The intravenous feeding of an infant, commonly a very premature infant, with a solution of amino acids, glucose, electrolytes, and vitamins.

Hyperosmolar   A fluid that is of higher osmotic pressure than the reference fluid. Elemental formulas are hyperosmolar; breastmilk is iso-osmolar with human serum.

Hyper-prolactinemia   Higher than normal prolactin levels, which may result in spontaneous breastmilk production and amenorrhea. Causes include pituitary tumors and some pharamaceuticals. See *also*: Prolactin.

Hypothalamus   A gland which controls postpartum serum prolactin levels through release of dopamine. Inhibition of dopamine permits the release of prolactin, which controls the secretion of milk.

Immunity, active   Immunity conferred by the production of antibodies by one's own immune system.

Immunity, passive   Immunity conferred on an infant by antibodies manufactured by the mother and passed to the infant transplacentally or in breastmilk. Passive immunity is temporary but very important to the young infant.

Immunoassay   Any method for the quantitative determination of chemical substances which uses the highly specific binding between antigen or hapten and homologous antibodies. E.g., radioimmunoassay, enzyme immunoassay, and fluoroimmunoassay.

Immunogen   A substance which stimulates the body to form antibodies. *See also*: Antigen.

Immunoglobulin   Proteins produced by plasma cells in response to an immunogen. The five types are IgG, IgA, IgM, IgE, and IgD. IgG is transferred in utero and provides passive immunity to infections to which the mother is immune; IgA is the principal immunoglobulin in colostrum and mature milk; IgM is produced by the neonate soon after birth and is also contained in breastmilk. *See also*: Non-casein protein.

Incubation period   The period between exposure to infectious pathogens and the first signs of illness.

Infection control   Practices–in hospitals formalized by protocols–which reduce the chance that infection will be spread between patients or between patients and staff. Handwashing and wearing of rubber gloves are two such practices.

International Code of Marketing of Breast-Milk Substitutes   A set of resolutions which regulate the marketing and distribution of any fluid intended to replace breastmilk, certain devices used to feed such fluids, and the role of health-care workers who advise on infant feeding. Developed by members of a joint commission convened in 1979 by WHO and UNICEF, it was approved in 1981 by members of the World Health Organization (only the United States dissented). Intended as a voluntary model which could be incorporated into the legal code of individual nations in order to enhance national efforts to promote breastfeeding. Also referred to as the "WHO Code" or the "WHO/UNICEF Code."

Intracellula   Occurring within cells. Viruses live within other cells during part of their reproductive lives. Although virus within cells may be passed to the infant in breastmilk, other cells in breastmilk enhance the destruction of these infected cells.

Intrauterine   Within the uterus; in utero.

Intrauterine growth rate   The normal rate of weight gain of a fetus. It is considered by many, but not all, physicians to be the ideal growth rate for premature infants.

Lactase   Enzyme needed to convert lactose to simple sugars usable by the infant. Present from birth in the intestinal mucosa, its activity diminishes after weaning.

Lactase deficiency   See: Lactose intolerance.

Lactiferous ducts   Milk ducts. Fifteen to 24 tubes which collect milk from the smaller ductules and carry it to the nipple. They appear similar to stems on a bunch of grapes, the alveoli being the "grapes." The ducts open into nipple pores.

Lactiferous sinuses   Dilations in the lactiferous ducts under the areola which act as small milk reservoirs. In order to nurse effectively, an infant must take enough breast into his mouth to be able to strip milk from these sinuses.

Lactobacillus bifidus   Principal bacillus in the intestinal flora of breastfed infants. Low intestinal pH (5-6) of fully breastfed infants discourages the colonization of *Streptococcus faecalis, Bacteroides sp.* and *E. coli*, which are common in feces of infants fed cow's-milk-based infant milks.

Lactoengineering   The process of fortifying human milk with nutrients derived from other batches of human milk, especially protein, calcium, and phosphorus, in order to meet the special nutritional needs of very low-birth-weight infants. *See also*: Human milk fortifiers.

Lactoferrin   A protein which is an important immunological component of human milk. It binds iron in the intestinal tract, thus denying it to bacteria which require iron to survive. Exogenous iron may upset this balance. *See also*: Non-casein protein.

Lactogenesis   The initiation of milk secretion. The initial synthesis of milk components which begins late in pregnancy may be termed lactogenesis I; the onset of copious milk production two or three days postpartum may be termed lactogenesis II.

Lactose intolerance   The manifestation of lactase deficiency; the inability of the intestines to digest lactose, the principal carbohydrate in human milk. More common beyond early childhood because of diminished activity of intestinal lactase, especially in cultures which do not use milk or milk products as foods after early childhood.

Lactose   The principal carbohydrate in human milk–about 4% of colostrum and 7% of mature milk. A disaccharide, it metabolizes readily to glucose, which is used for energy, and galactose, which assists lipids that are laid down in the brain. Lactose also enhances calcium absorption, thus helping prevent rickets in the breastfed infant, and it inhibits the growth of pathogens in the breastfed infant's intestine.

Larynx   The region at the upper end of the trachea (windpipe) through which the voice is produced. In the infant, the larynx lies close to the base of the tongue; during swallowing it rises and is closed off by the epiglottis.

Lesion   Circumscribed area of injured or diseased skin.

Let-down   The milk-ejection reflex. Caused by contraction of myoepithelial cells surrounding the alveoli in which milk is secreted. It is under the control of oxytocin released during nipple stimulation and sometimes of psychological influences.

Leukocytes   Living cells, including macrophages and lymphocytes, which inhabit breastmilk and combat infection.

Licensure   The process whereby an agency of state government grants permission to an individual, who is accountable for the practice of a profession, to engage in that profession. The corollary of licensure is that unlicensed individuals are prohibited from legally practicing licensed professions. The purpose of licensure is to protect the public by ensuring professional competence.

Ligand   A small molecule that binds specifically to a larger molecule. E.g., the binding of an antigen to an antibody, or a hormone to a receptor.

Lipase   Enzyme which aids the digesiton of milk fats by reducing them to a fine emulsion.

Low-birth-weight   Term applied to infants weighing less than 2500 gm at birth.

Lymphadenopathy   Abnormal swelling of lymph nodes.

Lymphocyte   A mature leukocyte; a lymph cell which is bactericidal.

Lyophilization   A process of rapid freeze drying of a fluid under a high vacuum. This process is used on human milk to obtain nutrient fractions used to fortify expressed human milk.

Lysozyme   Enzyme in breastmilk which is active against E. *coli* and *Salmonella*. *See also*: Non-casein protein.

Mammary bud   A clump of embryonic epithelial cells formed along the mammary ridge, which extend into the underlying mesenchyme. It develops about 49 days postconception. From this bud sprout the precursors of the milk ducts.

Mammary ridge   Milk line. The linear thickening of epithelial cells to each side of the midline of the embryo. Develops during weeks five through eight. Later this ridge differentiates into breast and nipple tissue.

Mandible   The lower jaw. Strong, rhythmic closing of the mandible during breastfeeding drives the compression of the lacteriferous sinuses, one component of the infant's milking process.

Mature milk   Breast milk commonly produced after about two weeks postpartum and containing no admixture of colostrum. It is higher in lactose, fat, and water-soluble vitamins. Its exact composition varies in response to infant needs.

Median   The middle number in a series of numbers; the number on either side of which exist an equal amount of numbers.

Mesenchyme   The embryonic mesoderm.

Mitosis   A type of cell division in which each daughter cell contains the same DNA as the parent cell.

Morbidity   The number of ill persons or instances of a disease in a specific population.

Mortality   The number of deaths in a specific population.

Mucocutaneous   Involving both mucous membranes and skin. Herpes blisters, for example, can form on both sites.

Multiparous   A woman who has carried two or more pregnancies to viability.

Myelination   The process by which conducting nerve fibers develop a protective fatty sheath. The long-chain polyunsaturated fats which are important to myelination are abundant in human milk; they are much less abundant in cow's milk or cow's-milk-based infant milks. Loss of myelin is a characteristic of the disease multiple sclerosis.

Myoepithelial cells   Contractile cells. In the breast these cells surround the milk-secreting alveoli; their contraction forces milk into the milk ducts. When many of these cells contract at the same time a "let-down" occurs. *See also*: let-down.

Necrotizing enterocolitis   Inflammation of the intestinal tract which may cause tissue to die. Premature infants not receiving human milk are at markedly greater risk for this serious complication of premature birth.

Neurotransmitter   A chemical which is selectively released from a nerve terminal by an action potential and then interacts with a specific receptor on an adjacent structure to produce a specific physiologic response.

Nipple   Cylindrical pigmented protuberance on the breast into which the lactiferous ducts open. The human nipple contains 15 to 20 nipple pores through which milk flows. The mammary papilla.

Nipple, inverted   A nipple which is retracted into the breast both when at rest and when stimulated.

Non-casein protein   The protein in the whey portion of milk. Non-casein proteins in human milk include alphalactalbumin, serum albumin, lactoferrin, immunoglobulins, and lysozyme.

Non-Governmental Organization (NGO)   Title conferred by UNICEF on private organizations which command expertise valuable to UNICEF; such organizations are permitted to comment on and attempt to influence UNICEF activities. La Leche League International and the International Lactation Consultant Association are NGOs.

Nonprotein nitrogen (NPN)   About one-fourth of the total nitrogen in human milk is derived from sources, such as urea, other than protein. NPN contains several free amino acids, including leucine, valine, and threonine, which are essential in the young infant's diet because he cannot yet manufacture them.

Nutriment   Any nourishing substance.

Oligosaccharide   Carbohydrate, comprised of a few monosaccharides, present in human milk. Some oligosaccharides promote the growth of Lactobacillus *bifidus*, thus increasing intestinal acidity, which discourages the growth of intestinal pathogens.

Oral rehydration therapy (ORT)   The administration by mouth of a solution of water, salt, and sugar in order to replace body fluids lost during severe diarrhea. The proportions of elements in an oral rehydration solution are essentially the same as they are in breastmilk. Artificially fed infants are much more susceptible than those who are breastfed to the diarrhea which may lead to severe dehyration and the need for ORT.

Oxytocin   A lactogenic hormone produced in the posterior pituitary gland. It is released during suckling (or other nipple stimulation) and causes ejection of milk as well as uterine contractions.

Palate, hard   The hard, anterior roof of the mouth. A suckling infant uses his tongue to compress breast tissue against the hard palate.

Palate, soft   The soft, posterior roof of the mouth, which lies between the hard palate and the throat. It rises during swallowing to close off nasal passages. The velum.

Parenchyma   The functional parts of an organ. In the breast, the parenchyma include the mammary ducts, lobes, and alveoli.

Parenteral   Introduction of fluids, nutrients or drugs into the body by any avenue other than the digestive tract.

Pasteurization   The heating of milk to destroy pathogens. Milk banks commonly heat donor milk to 56° for 30 minutes.

Pathogen   Substance or organism capable of producing illness.

Peristalsis   Involuntary, rhythmic, wave-like action. Commonly thought of in relation to food and waste products moving along the gastrointestinal tract. In order to strip milk from the breast, an infant's tongue utilizes a peristaltic motion which begins at the tip of the tongue and progresses towards the back of the mouth.

Pharynx   The muscular tube at the rear of the mouth, through which nasal air travels to the larynx and food from the mouth travels to the esophagus. During infant feeding, contraction of pharyngeal muscles moves a bolus of fluid into the esophagus.

Pituitary   An endocrine gland at the base of the brain which secretes several hormones. Prolactin, which is essential for production of milk, is secreted by the anterior lobe; oxytocin, which is essential for milk let-down, is secreted by the posterior lobe.

Placenta   The intrauterine organ that transfers nutrients from the mother to the fetus. The expulsion of the placenta at birth causes an abrupt drop in estrogen and progesterone, which in turn permits the secretion of milk.

Polymastia   The presence of more than two breasts. These additional structures, which usually contain only a small amount of glandular tissue, may occur anywhere along the milk line from axilla to groin.

Premature infant   One born before 37 weeks gestational age, regardless of birth weight.

Primary infection   The first incidence of illness after exposure to a pathogen.

Primiparous   A woman who has carried one pregnancy to viability.

Progesterone   Hormone produced by the corpus luteum and placenta which maintains a pregnancy and helps develop the mammary alveoli.

Prolactin   Hormone which is produced in the anterior pituitary gland. It stimulates development of the breast and controls milk synthesis. Normal concentrations are 10-25 ng/ml in a nonpregnant woman; 200-400 ng/ml at birth.

Prone   Lying on one's stomach.

Respiratory syncytial virus (RSV)   Organism causing a respiratory illness; breastfed infants are at less risk for this illness.

Rickets   Abnormal calcification of the bones and changes in growth plates which lead to soft or weak bones. Rarely seen in breastfed children; exceptions include those not exposed to the sun.

Rotavirus   A class of viruses which are a major cause of diarrheal illness leading to hospitalization of infants. Breastfed infants are at less risk for illness caused by this organism.

Rugae   Corrugations on the hard palate behind the gum ridge, which help the infant to retain a grasp on the breast during suckling.

Sebaceous glands   Glands which secrete oil. Those on the areola are called tubercules of Montgomery. The oil they secrete is presumed to lubricate and provide bacteriostatic protection to the areola.

Secretory IgA   An immunoglobulin abundant in human milk which is of immense value to the neonate. It is synthesized and stored in the breast; after ingestion by the infant it blocks adhesion of pathogens to the intestinal mucosa.

Secretory immune system   The system which produces specific antibodies or thymus-influenced lymphocytes in response to specific antigens.

Sepsis   The presence of bacteria in fluid or tissue.

Seroconvert   For serum to show the presence of a factor which previously has been absent, or the reverse. When antibodies to an infecting agent, such as cytomegalovirus, become present the person is said to have seroconverted.

Serological tests   Tests performed on blood samples to ascertain the presence or absence of pathogens.

Seronegative   Serum which does not demonstrate the presence of a factor tested for; "tests negative."

Seropositive   Serum which demonstrates the presence of a factor test for; "test positive."

Serum   Clear fluid portion of blood which remains after coagulation.

Serum albumin   A protein in serum. See also: Non-casein protein.

Smooth muscle   The type of muscle which provides the erectile tissue in the nipple and areola.

Somatic   Pertaining to the body, especially nonreproductive tissue.

Spontaneous lactation   Secretion and release of milk unrelated to a pregnancy or to nipple stimulation intended to stimulate milk production.

Suck, Suckle   Used in this textbook interchangeably to mean the baby's milking action at the breast. In traditional usage, a baby at the breast "sucked," while a mother "suckled."

Sucking, non-nutritive   Sucking not at the breast–e.g., as on a pacifier or on baby's own tongue. Or, sucking at the breast characterized by alternating brief sucks and long rest periods during minimal milk flow. However, insofar as any milk is transferred, even this latter pattern of sucking may in fact be nutritive. See also: Sucking, nutritive .

Sucking, nutritive   Steady rhythmic sucking during full, continuous milk flow. Insofar as any milk is transferred, other sucking patterns also may be nutritive. *See also*: Sucking, non-nutritive.

Symbiosis   The intimate association of two different kinds of organisms. The breastfeeding dyad is considered by many to exemplify a mutually beneficial symbiosis.

Systemic immune system   The nonspecific immune responses of the body.

T-cells   Any of several kinds of thymic lymphoid cells or lymphocytes which help regulate cellular immune response. A subset of these cells (T4-cells) are preferentially attacked by Human Immunodeficiency Virus.

Teleological   Describing the belief that all events are directed toward some ultimate purpose.

Thrombocytopenia   Low levels of platelets in blood.

TORCH   Acronym for organisms which can damage the fetus: Toxoplasmosis, Rubella, Cytomegalovirus, Herpes simplex.

Tracheoesophageal fistula (T-E fistula)   An abnormal opening between the trachea and esophagus; this congenital malformation occurs in about 1:3000 births. T-E fistula may cause a neonate to aspirate fluids. Colostrum, a physiologic fluid, is much less irritating to the lungs than water, glucose water, or artificial infant milks.

Transcutaneous bilimeter   A device which estimates bilirubin concentrations in the blood by measuring intensity of yellowish skin coloration.

Transitional milk   Breast fluid of continuously varying composition produced in the first two- to-three weeks postpartum as colostrum decreases and milk production increases.

Transplacental   Transferred from mother to fetus through the placenta. Nutrients and certain immunoglobulins are, and some infections may also be, transferred to the fetus transplacentally.

United Nations Childrens' Fund (UNICEF)   Originally established in 1946 as the United Nations International Childrens' Emergency Fund. An agency of the United Nations charged with protecting the lives of children and enabling them to lead fuller lives. It assists member nations in providing health care, safe water, sanitation, nutrition, housing, education, and training to accomplish these goals.

Universal precautions   Guidelines for infection control based on the assumption that every person receiving health care carries an infection which can be transmitted by blood, body fluids, or genital secretions.

Vaccine   An infectious agent, or derivatives of one, given to a person so that his immune system will produce antibodies to that infection without a preceding illness.

Vertical transmission   Transmission of infection from mother to child transplacentally or through breastmilk.

Very low birth weight   Term applied to infants weighing less than 1500 gm at birth.

Virus   Very small organisms which rely on material in invaded cells to reproduce. Viruses identified in breastmilk include cytomegalovirus, Herpes zoster and *Herpes simplex*, hepatitis, and rubella.

Water soluble vitamins   The B vitamins and vitamin C; pantothenic acid, biotin, and folate. These vitamins are present in serum; concentrations in breastmilk approximate those in serum. Concentrations reflect current maternal diet more directly than do fat-soluble vitamins (A, D, E, K).

Wet nurses   Women who breastfeed for pay infants who are not their own.

Whey   The liquid left after curds are separated from milk. Alphalactalbumin and lactoferrin are the principal whey proteins. Because human milk has a whey-to-casein ratio of about 65:35, it froms soft, easily digested curds in the infant stomach. See *also*: Casein, non-casein protein.

Witch's milk   Colostrum, formed under the influence of maternal hormones, which may be expressed from temporarily enlarged mammary tissue in the neonate's breasts.

World Health Organization (WHO)   An agency of the United Nations charged with planning and coordinating global health care and assisting member nations to combat disease and train health workers.

Xeropthalmia   Disease of the eyes caused by vitamin-A deficiency; it is endemic in parts of Africa. Human milk is a preventive.

MEDICAL ABBREVIATIONS USED THROUGHOUT

Breastfeeding and Human Lactation

>	greater than
<	less than
=	equal to
ā	before
ab	abortion
ABC	alternative birthing center
abd	abdomen
ABG	arterial blood gases
AIDS	Acquired Immunodeficiency Syndrome
BBT	basal body temperature
Bf	breastfed/breastfeeding
B/P	blood pressure
BPD	bronchopulmonary dysplasia
BSE	breast self examination
BUN	blood urea nitrogen
C	centigrade
c̄	with
CA	cancer
Ca	calcium
cal	calorie
CHD	congenital heart disease
CBC	complete blood count
cc	cubic centimeter
CMV	cytomegalovirus
CNS	central nervous system
CPAP	continuous positive airway pressure
C&S	culture and sensitivity
c/sec	cesarean birth

CNM	Certified nurse midwife
CSF	cerebral spinal fluid
CVA	cardiovascular accident
CVP	central venous pressure
D5W	5% dextrose in water
D&C	dilation and curettage
D/C	discharge
dc	discontinue
DR	delivery room
DRG	diagnostic related groups
dx	diagnosis
ECG	electrocardiogram
EDC	estimated date of confinement (due date)
EDD	estimated date of delivery
EEG	electroencephalogram
epis	episiotomy
EENT	eyes, ears, nose, throat
EFM	electronic fetal monitoring
ER	emergency room
ET	endotracheal tube
FAS	fetal alcohol syndrome
FBD	fibrocystic breast disease
FBS	fasting blood sugar
FLK	funny looking kid
FSH	follicular stimulating hormone
FTT	failure to thrive
FUO	fever of unknown origin
GDM	gestational diabetes mellitus
GI	gastrointestinal
gm	gram
gr	grain
grav	gravida (number of pregnancies)
GU	genitourinary
GYN	gynecology
hct	hematocrit
Hg	mercury
H&P	history and physical
ht	height
hx	history

IDDM	Insulin-dependent diabetes mellitus
IUGR	intrauterine growth retardation
IM	intramuscular
I&O	intake and output
IUD	intrauterine device
IV	intravenous
JCAH	Joint Commission on the Accreditation of Hospitals
Kg	kilogram
L	liter
Ⓛ	left
lab	laboratory
LC	lactation consultant
LGA	large for gestational age
LMP	last menstrual period
Mcg	microgram
mec	meconium
med	medication
mg	milligram
ml	milliliter
NANDA	North American Nursing Diagnosis Association
NEC	necrotizing enterocolitis
n/g	nasogastric
NPO	nothing by mouth
nsg	nursing (breastfeeding)
Ø	no, none
OB	obstetrical
OT	occupational therapy
OTC	over the counter
oz	ounce
p̄	after
para	number of living children
pc	after meals (refers to *post cibum*)
PDA	patent ductus arteriosus
peri	perineal
ph	degree of acidity/alkalinity
PID	pelvic inflammatory disease
PIH	pregnancy-induced hypertension

PKU	phenylketonuria
po	by mouth
prn	as needed
PT	physical therapist
q	every, each
qd	every day
qid	4 times/day
℞	right
RBC	red blood cell
RDA	recommended dietary allowances
RDS	respiratory distress syndrome
REM	rapid eye movement
Rh	Rhesus blood factor
R/O	rule out
Rx	medication/prescription
s̄	without
SGA	small for gestational age
SIDS	sudden infant death syndrome
SOAP	subjective data, objective data, analysis, plan
staph	staphylococcus
STD	sexually transmitted disease
strep	streptococcus
tid	3 times/day
u/a	urinalysis
URI	upper respiratory infection
UTI	urinary tract infection
VBAC	vaginal birth after cesarean
WBC	white blood cell
WIC	Special Supplemental Food Program for Women, Infants, and Children